Eleanor's Gift

*Hospice Stories about
Loving, Caring and Dying*

Patricia Spencer Blunt

BeKind Publishers
Midlothian, Virginia

Eleanor's Gift

Hospice Stories about
Loving, Caring and Dying

ISBN: 0-9749057-0-4   US $15.95

Library of Congress Control Number: 2002108905

BeKind Publishers
Midlothian, Virginia 23114

Original Version Edited and Printed by
Raj Publishing, Inc., Jacksonville, Florida

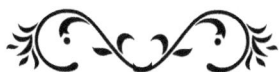

"Those who don't know how to weep with their whole heart don't know how to laugh either."

—-Golda Meir

Acknowledgments

A Note from the Editor...

F rom the beginning, Patty and I have been committed to making this a project with no rules and only proceeding when the way is open and easy. When the task became grueling, we put it away for a while. When the synchronicity kicked in and everything seemed to flow naturally, we moved forward.

Realizing that it is generally the author who writes an acknowledgement, we determined not to let that stop us in writing as many "thank you's" in as many ways as we felt necessary to complete the task. We both had tremendous support from so many people and wanted to share our gratitude.

Our original publisher, Ted, was a tremendous resource in so many ways — encouraging, making recommendations, being open and adaptable to changes, and just being available. Without Mary, our transcriptionist, the words would never have made it from Patty's tape recorder to my computer, so there would have been no book.

My friend and author, Dr. Margee Howe-Bugbee, was my encourager. She shared her knowledge of the book world, brainstormed titles and strategies, dragged me to writing seminars and book signings, and generally made me believe we could actually create and market this book.

My family and so many other friends were supportive in every possible way; it would be difficult to name them all. Most importantly, I am indebted to Patty for sharing this experience with me. I have grown mentally and spiritually because of whom she is and what she gives to others.

— K. Mixson

Acknowledgments

A Note from the Author...

$\mathcal{I}$f I thanked all the people who helped with this book, it would be another book. But first I want to thank God for making all of this possible and for the help He provided. Second, of course, Eleanor for starting it all for my education. And Cindy....

I would especially like to thank the heroes in this world. These are the patient caregivers I have worked with, all of the families, and the patients themselves.

Without my goddess friends, none of this would have happened. This book would never have been written. Thanks to:

Kathy — my dear, dear friend, who provided editing and had all the business acumen. She is an absolute miracle.

Mary — I have never known anybody who could make things look so good on paper, dear, dear heart. She is a true friend who has helped me through many things.

Margee, who provided all the technical and moral support, and Walter, who provided knowledge and supported Margee. Their caring and friendship really bolstered us all through this process.

Especially, though, I want to thank my patients who have gone ahead, who taught me so much, who support me even now — that is Allan, Kitty, Rudy, and Richard.

I would like to thank David Prentice of Lightning Source and Olivia Cloud of Guardian Angel Communication Services in Nashville for helping me produce the revised edition of this book.

I also want to thank all of the people I have worked with at Hospice over the years. There are some people who mentored me without even knowing it: Dr. Skip Wilson, Dr. Meade, Dr. Joe, Dr. Fink, and Dr. Ted. Thank you all for being who you are, you have taught me so much. I'm grateful to the Equipment staff for being my friends and to the pharmacy for listening to my craziness and for getting patients the care they need.

And so many others...Sharon, Mary Ann, Trudy, Marilynn, Bonnie, Laurie, Jeff, Danny, Tweet, Lucy, Sally, Britt, Carol, Ken, Elaine, Randy, Lyn, Marie, Mary, M.H., Barbara, Ethel, Karen, E.J., Connie, Ruth, Beth, Judy, Cookie, Vickie, Alice, Jim, Brent, Angie, Mark, Dan, Barry, Christy, Amanda, Fred, Rich, Howard, Frank, Jackie, Suzi, Bob, Bertha, Bill, Tyler, and Toni.

I want to thank my parents, who taught me the concept of apostolic action and the meaning it gives to life. They have given me so much more than I can put into words.

My daughter, Cindy, who said that one statement that has helped me explain the concept of dying to people, which is that death is like "birth in reverse." She is teaching me how to let go and love.

Words cannot express my gratitude to my husband, Todd, for his support and encouragement of me and the work that God has given me to do.

I appreciate the incredible support we have received from total strangers who helped us along the way. To me, this is just further proof that there is a loving, kind, supportive God.

There are so many other anonymous people that I would love to thank by name. You know who you are, and I wish you all the very best.

I also want to thank in advance the people who are reading this. I hope you take your laughter and your tears and share them with others. Pass it on.

— Patricia Spencer Blunt Weatherford

Table of Contents

Preface

I have never had any desire to write a book. I was just a burned out Hospice nurse. One night, after a very hard day of nursing, I went to the pool, put on my mask, and started swimming. I was crying under water, saying, "God, I can't do this any more. You called me into Hospice and I don't want to leave without You calling me out. Please call me out!"

I heard Him (in an inaudible but distinct voice) say, "Patty, you have to share your knowledge with people. There are things my people need to know."

I insisted, "I'll write it all down later, I promise."

He said, "Hon, if I call you out, you won't remember. Get it on paper now...write a book."

I said, "What! I can't write a book!" And I continued to argue with Him, giving all the excuses why I couldn't do this.

But God said, "You have done the things I have asked you to and I have given you the power to do them. This is no different."

"It IS different," I pleaded. "I've taken typing seven times and still can't type fast, and I have to work, too. I can't write something the public will read. And, by the way, what would I write?"

As I swam lap after lap in the pool, God gently told me... "I will help you."

And He proceeded to bring to my mind different people (patients) and families—people I had worked with in Hospice over the years. When I got home, I wrote down the names on a piece of paper. The book had begun!

In college I used to put my notes on tape, so I thought I could write if I could just put it all on tape. But then I would have the problem of typing it up afterwards.

One day, while visiting one of my patients, I mentioned this "order" I had been given to Mary, the daughter of one of my patients. Over the next few visits she would ask me how the book was coming. After a couple of times, I confessed that the "darn typing" was the problem.

She just got excited. She is a medical transcriptionist and can type anything. She said she could take my tapes and type them up. She said she could even type from anyone's writing. I challenged her with my journal pages. When writing for my own eyes, my writing is not always easy to read. But when on a subsequent visit she handed me back my complete typed journal, I just cried. I thought, "God, You are putting this together!"

But a whole book? That would be a lot of work. To get me to accept her help, Mary assured me she would enjoy doing it.

I started telling the story of each patient on my list into my tape recorder and taking it to Mary. Each time I took her a tape, she would hand me an envelope of the typed up stories on diskette. The memory still brings tears to my eyes. My friend Mary was part of God's plan for the book, I am sure.

Another night I was relaying this miracle to Kathy, another friend. She just lit up and asked, "Do you have an editor yet?"

I said, "For heaven's sake, I don't even want to write this book. I haven't thought about getting an editor."

She asked, "Can I at least read it?"

I said, "Sure, but it probably won't make any sense."

Kathy laughed, and said, "I have always wanted to edit a book. I would be honored if you would let me do that."

I know when Kathy really wants to do something, so I said yes. It was so hard for me to accept more help. However, her enthusiasm was contagious.

So now the team was in place. It had now become "our book"— God's, Mary's, Kathy's and mine.

This is my first up-close-and-personal look at God orchestrating a team effort. He knew I couldn't do it alone, nor did I need to. This has been a life lesson for me. It really moves me to think that this higher power would love me so much, to give me two wonderful friends whom I love and care about. The gratitude I feel is over-whelming.

It is my hope…our hope…that something in the pages that follow will bless you.

— Patty

Please Note…

…that all of the names, except Eleanor's, have been changed in consideration for the families, and in some cases situations have been altered.

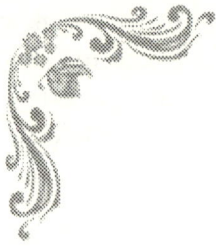

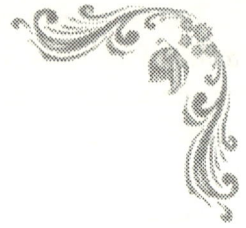

Chapter One

GIVE THANKS WHERE THANKS IS DUE

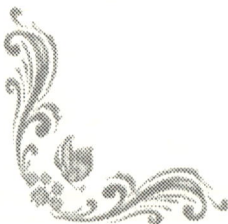

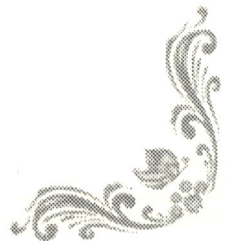

GIVE THANKS WHERE THANKS IS DUE

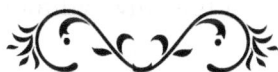

My dad looked at me with the eyes of a child—frustrated and tired. I said, "Dad, thank you so much for changing my diapers when I was little and thank you for sending me to college."

He looked at me and said, "I sent you to college?"

I touched his forehead and kissed him, and said, "Yeah, you did. Thank you so much."

Being a Hospice nurse, I deal with critical illness on a daily basis. However, I never really thought about this situation on a personal basis. I went to North Carolina to take care of my dad while he was recuperating from minor knee surgery. I ended up facing the possibility of going through his physical decline, and taking care of both him and my mother at the same time.

My dad went in the hospital for knee surgery on Monday the 24th of June. I had flown up from Florida to take care of him and help my mother. Dad wanted so much to come home after the surgery, because he was getting no rest in the hospital. The second night there, he had taken two sleeping pills and two pain pills, and ended up crawling out of bed and falling. I knew in my heart we needed to bring him home.

He was fine when he first got home, but then he started getting confused. He couldn't even stand up to use the walker. He couldn't get his arms and legs to work at the same time. Also, he would sit at the kitchen table, but could not feed himself. Just getting him to the table was a challenge, since he couldn't bend his knee due to the incision. It was horrible—so much confusion.

Both my parents were so stubborn that they would not allow me to order a bedside commode or a wheelchair. They had built this small handicap bathroom right off the kitchen in a little closet. There was a high potty with a handicap rail on the side. One day, both Dad and I got stuck with his walker in this tiny bathroom, unable to move. He had been constipated in the hospital, so I had given him Senokot S[1] and he ended up having an accident in his pants.

He looked at me and said, "I think I messed all over myself."

I said, "Well, Honey, I think you did, too, but it's not a big deal."

It was just unbelievable.

I had a flashback to when I first became a nurse and had asked my dad what he was going to do when he got older. He said, "Well, when I can't do everything for myself, I am just going to walk out into the sunset. I'll be darned if you are going to change my diaper!"

The next morning I truly thought he was declining. I said to my mom, "I need a wheelchair and bedside commode to take care of him. That is it!" I had not trusted my instincts and my education up to then. We had needed those things two days ago, and I had let them talk me out of it.

It really shook me how the whole scenario reminded me of my Hospice patients. That's when I became convinced that people who take care of their loved ones at home need some education. They need to know what to do, and when and how to do it. They need to know basic care: how to use a draw sheet, the importance of using plastic gloves, staying healthy, and staying close to the patient. They need to know how to transfer incapacitated people from wheelchair to bed or chair, and how to deal with a confused person.

It really made me realize how much people don't know when they are thrown into this situation. But I wouldn't have missed this experience for the world! I still didn't know what was going to happen, but I took care of him—and by this time Dad had no shame. I sat at the kitchen table admiring the beautiful rose garden he had planted. Then I gave him a bath and washed his feet. And I thought, this is an honor.

We called the neurologist to discuss our concerns about Dad's decline and his medication. Dad had knee replacement surgery the previous year and had recovered with no problems. However, he did not have Parkinson's disease then.

The neurologist thought the Sinemet[2], which Dad had been taking since being diagnosed with Parkinson's, could be reacting with some medication related to the knee surgery. He suggested we stop that medication for the time being. We were willing to try anything.

My parents have been married for a long time, but I had never realized that my "kick-butt" independent mother was so dependent on my dad. When he was so sick, her response was complete denial.

Once, when he was about to fall, I needed her help. I was trying to get his pants off without getting feces in his incision, and called to her for help. My mother sounded close by, so I am sure she heard me. But do you know what she did? She went to do laundry—laundry!! I thought, what's wrong with this picture?!

But that is how she responded to the stress. She was scared. I had people I could call and cry with, but she did not. My support network kept me out of denial and kept me functioning. However, she does have a really strong faith. She introduced me to God early in my life as the ultimate relationship (i.e., Friend, Father, Brother).

That night I went to a chapel near my parents' house, and cried and cried. I thought, God, I can't do this. You can't take my dad. He is so young and he has gone through so much… I realized that my family was going through all the things my Hospice families go through—it all connected. While talking to God, I realized I felt unworthy to take care of my dad. Then I thought of how far God had brought me and what He had given me. It all made sense, and I knew I could do it. So I accepted it. I always do best when I accept the worst possible thing that can happen.

When I left the chapel, I was cried out and exhausted. But I had a clear understanding that whatever God wanted me to do, He would give me the power to do it. He had promised me His spirit.

When I got home, I got my dad on his feet. He could use his walker and his coordination was back. I thought—once again, I accept whatever is going to happen, and then it changes. It is incredible. You have to let go of what you want to happen. I think I have tried so insincerely to "let go" for so long, just to get what I wanted—but this taught me a lesson.

I never appreciated all the skills that I have acquired until this experience. I have done things I didn't know I could do, and God filled in the blanks. With all we went through, my dad never hurt himself—not once. When I resigned myself and just said, "Okay, God, I accept whatever will happen," then my dad was better. He was so much better.

Life is very fragile. Please tell the people you love that you love them. I told my dad that I loved him that night. During the time he was confused; he said, "Love you too, Hon." However, when his medication was corrected and he was himself again, he gave no response. But I think that was okay. It is not important what my parents say or don't say, but it IS important that they know I love them. They have to know that and I need to tell them often.

I went back to the chapel to give credit where credit was due. I just sat there in the quiet. God, You are amazing—just amazing! Thank You... thank You.

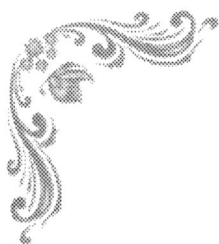

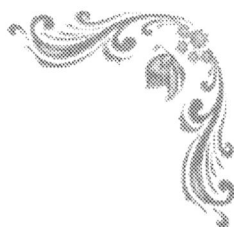

Chapter Two

A HOSPICE NURSE

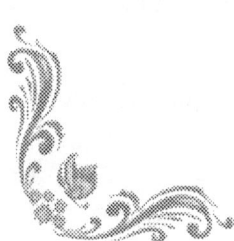

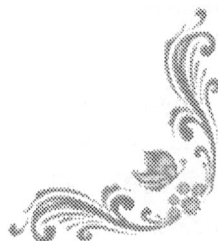

A HOSPICE NURSE

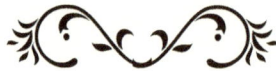

*don't think anybody wakes up one morning and says, "Yes, I want to be a Hospice nurse." Maybe an ICU nurse. Maybe they've seen "ER" on television. But I believe with all my heart that God has to choose people to work in Hospice. Number one reason—death is something that all of us will experience, yet it is one of the things that people fear most—outside of public speaking, of course.

In my prayer time, as the time comes to close the Hospice nursing chapter of my life, I feel it is my responsibility to pass on the knowledge I have gained through different situations experienced and how I got into Hospice.

Eleanor was the first person to introduce me to God in skin. She loved me when I was an unlovable teenager. She was married to a minister, whom I never met. She had the best sense of humor. She just laughed at everything.

Eleanor knew everything about me and yet never judged. She was a deaconess in the church, an elder, and just…light personified. She was hysterically funny, and she befriended me at a time when I really needed a friend.

Eleanor lived in North Carolina and I met her when I was 16 years old. She always called me "Trail Boss" after we hiked up to Mt. Piscah together. That was my first encounter with near death.

At the time she was probably in her late 70's. We got to the top of this mountain. A cold rain was falling. I turned to talk to her and she looked like she was dying. I thought, God, what will happen? What do I do with a woman in her late 70's who dies on top of a mountain? Do I drag the body down the mountain all by myself? Or, do I go down the mountain and tell somebody she's up there? She was not looking good. But we stayed up there for a while until she was better, and we did indeed make it back down the mountain. It was a close call.

I later went back to Florida and, several years later, God called me to go to nursing school. My business had failed and I needed a way to support my child and myself.

During the last semester of nursing school, Eleanor called me and said, "Are you sitting down?"

I said, "Yeah."

She said, "I now know how God is going to get me out of my body." She was a very spiritual woman, but she always put things into terms I could understand. She said, "I've been diagnosed with liver cancer, and I thought that since you are in the medical field that you would like to be a part of it. Would you?"

So, being in school and kind of brain dead, I said, "Why, of course!"

I stayed in contact with her by phone, and also through other people I knew in North Carolina. Eventually, Eleanor was transferred to an inpatient Hospice unit, meaning she was in the hospital. This happened in just three months.

Now this woman, before she was diagnosed, had won an award in the Senior Olympics. She was 87 years old and had cancer. To the best of my knowledge, she never drank anything alcoholic. She was just so healthy. She told me she always considered the spiritual retreats that she attended as "cramming for her finals." She was just a hoot. I knew she was prepared for her finals.

I found out that she was in the Hospice unit as I was taking my final exams in nursing school. I called her Hospice nurse in North Carolina and asked, "When should I come?"

She said, "I can't tell you that. She is not responding. She is not eating. She is not drinking. But you pray about it."

So I did. And that's what I have learned to say when families ask me, "When is my family member going to die? When should I come?" I always refer them back to what this Hospice nurse told me, and that is—go if you want to talk to the person while they are still lucid. If that is not part of your agenda, then go whenever. But if that is your main objective, go now.

I have also transferred that to my life. I tell people how I feel about them before I leave, because I have learned this in Hospice, from seeing family members who don't tell people and later regret it. Life is very short—very short.

I prayed about the situation with Eleanor, and I kept getting "Friday... Friday... " in my mind. My last exam was on Wednesday, and I told my professor (who knew about the situation) that I was going to drive up to see Eleanor. Before I left, she said, "I hope she recognizes you."

It was odd, because that same professor always gave me the patients that were dying when I was a nursing student. It was just part of what I did best. And yet I hated shots. I am not really a "nurse-type" personality. But I could handle dying people. It didn't bother me at all, because to me dying is just a part of life. There is a scripture that says we are "Absent from the body, present with the Lord."[3] I believe that.

So I drove up to North Carolina on Thursday and went to my parents' house. Next morning I drove over to Mission Hospital. A nurse met me at the elevator and asked, "Are you Patty?" When I said I was, she took me by the hand and led me into the room where two women—one I knew and one a stranger—were sitting by Eleanor's bed. Eleanor was wide-eyed, mouth open, and she was Cheyne-Stoking. That's what I call the "death breath."

I sat down, and Eleanor struggled to mouth the words, "Can you handle this?" in between breaths. She kept grabbing the Kleenex and became irritated. I realized she was trying to stuff Kleenex in my pocket—this person who was dying was so concerned for me.

By this time we were all crying. How long could she hang on like this? Was I going to be sitting on the side of the bed for days? The nurses kept saying, "We don't know what she's hanging on for. We told her that you were coming today. We felt she was waiting for you to get here."

Eleanor had made a statement on that first phone call when she asked if I wanted to be part of this dying process of hers. She said, "I think this is for your education." I didn't understand what she was saying until much later, after I got into Hospice work. For my education? I'd never had anybody do anything for my education, much less die!

So there we were in Eleanor's room, and Eleanor got a real strange look. We sang three hymns to her. I believe they were "How Great Thou Art," "Amazing Grace," and something else I can't remember now. I was just crying and crying.

As soon as I had surrendered to the fact that I might be sitting on the side of the bed for a long time, Eleanor took a long breath and her breathing started slowing down. She seemed to be holding her breath. Her eyes remained open, but she was not looking at any of us.

Suddenly, she got this full, knowing, loving look in her eyes and a presence came into the room. It was a thick, loving, peaceful, warm presence. Imagine being chilled, and then all of a sudden someone puts a warm blanket on top of you.

This presence saturated the room.

Without being able to physically see it, but with some kind of inner vision, I saw God asking Eleanor, "Are you ready to go?"

And she replied, "Yes."

I could see it! In my mind's eye I could see it. Then the presence left, but it left a thin film of that peace.

It was really weird and I was sobbing with so many emotions. I realized that her spirit was gone. I wasn't aware of anything else. About five minutes later a little pink lady, a volunteer, walked into the room.

Eleanor was lying there dead with her eyes open, and this little lady said to Eleanor, "Is there anything I can do for you, Honey?"

The three of us just turned around and looked at this little pink lady, not wanting to startle her. I said, "I don't think that she needs anything just now, but thank you so much."

After she left we started laughing and laughing. We laughed as if there were no tomorrow! Then we were crying again, and knowing the presence of God. It was all the presence of God. I truly think that is the first time that I understood that we are only one-third physical body. Our bodies are just a shell where our spirit resides.

There is a presence that is more wonderful than anything I have ever felt on earth. It came to that room that day, and Eleanor left with it. It was the God she kept telling me about and introducing me to, and that she served. It was the essence of peace. Though I am not a religious person, it was a faith builder, and it touched my spirit.

I have shared that story with those families who are so encrusted in the fact that the body is dying. The physical body is dying, and that is so important to them. Yes, it is important that the body is comfortable as it dies, but I think that is why I took to Hospice so readily, because I know the truth. And the truth definitely set me free—to work with Hospice.

But Hospice was not yet in the picture for me as a nurse. I graduated from nursing school and went to the Med/Surg[4] floor for my year of interning. They call it the "dump floor" in the hospital. I found that I hated nursing. Oh my gosh, it was so horrible—the IVs, the blood, the bandages! I worked nights for about a year, went to critical care, did everything I could to fill up my resume.

One day I went to a friend who was the director of nursing at Hospice and said, "You know, I can't stand this nursing. I just hate it."

She said, "Well, have you thought about Hospice nursing?"

I thought—get a grip! I had completely blanked out the whole event with Eleanor. I said, "Get serious—Hospice?"

One month later, I called her and said, "Could I just go follow one of your nurses around one day and see what it's like?"

She said, "Sure!"

So I did.

I got a speeding ticket that day because I followed that nurse everywhere. One of these nurses that go clear to "Egypt" for all of her homes and families. Every home was located out in the "boonies." But I watched what she did, and I went back to the hospital thinking—ah, that's not for me.

Another month went by. I was totally sick of working in the hospital—of people being referred to as a body part or a diagnosis. It was not "Mr. Smith in Room 403," but "the dialysis in 403." People were referred to as disease processes—I had just had it!

I called the Hospice director of nursing—anything had to be better than this.

She said, "Well, I am interviewing today, come on in. I also want you to interview with some people that don't know that we know each other."

So I did.

One woman who interviewed me, asked, "Why are you here?"

I told her the truth. I said, "God led me to this, and I am really unhappy working in the hospitals."

I walked out of there thinking—that's the dumbest thing you could ever say to someone. I got home with this killer headache and lay down on the bed.

I got a call about 20 minutes later from my director friend. She said, "You have the job, if you want it. How soon can you come in?"

I said, "I need to give two weeks notice."

She said, "I would expect nothing less."

So I went to work for Hospice.

During the orientation, seeing patients with other nurses was exciting. I loved it. I thought—YES, this is the kind of nursing I have been looking for! It wasn't even like nursing to me.

My orientation was supposed to take about five weeks. At the end of two weeks, however, my boss said, "You're going to start a little bit earlier. One of the nurses just resigned, so you'll be starting in a week. You will be taking over her patient load."

I was oriented very quickly. One nurse gave me "Signs and Symptoms of the Dying Process"—bless her heart. This is the little pamphlet that we give out to patients and their families. She said to read it and be able to explain it.

My mentors were excellent. I had a boss who answered my questions whenever I called—and I called a lot. It just all made sense to me. I didn't feel like I knew what I was doing for about a year. But the actual work—going into people's homes and dealing with the dying process—it was just like a "duck in water" for me. It was the most natural thing to talk about, to teach, to think about—and I have seen some incredible things over the past six years.

This kind of work has affected my life in a way I hope to express clearly. I hope this knowledge that I've gathered will be useful, because I have loved this work. I hope this will help someone, whether a Hospice nurse or a family member of a Hospice patient, or maybe a person just reading about this somewhat "taboo" subject. This work makes you deal with your own mortality and the actual dying process.

Once, I was sitting with a little lady who was living in her daughter's trailer. This lady had a "gazillion" academic degrees and was a college professor. She was loved by so many people, except her own family. Her family thought she was a real pain in the butt. But since she was family, they had her staying in their house.

She had started dying. She sat in this little room, not watching the TV, which was on. I would look at her while she was sleeping, and think—could I handle being her? Having a huge life behind me. Being an important and respected person. Knowing I had done all these important things, and now at the end of my life I was spending so much time alone. My thought was—I had best get my affairs in order!

This prompted me to do a lot of things. I called my mom and said, "Hey, I want to see the Grand Canyon before I die. Let's go." And we went. I told my family things that, if I thought they were going to live forever, I would probably never have shared with them. Whenever I would leave my friends, I was very expressive, because I saw people dying every day.

Working through their own death is very frightening for a lot of people—but what an opportunity.

That is how I got into Hospice. I have grown immensely, and can still remember writing years ago that I wanted to serve a purpose. I wanted to make a difference. And whenever I get discouraged, I affirm that, yes, as a Hospice nurse I am making a difference. Because what you say and do in this occupation affects people's lives.

I've seen God in so many different ways. I have seen the results of His actions. I've seen His spirit work through people, and I've seen Him come always at the perfect time to release someone's spirit from their body.

I hope that this helps whoever is reading this, because it is my time to come out of Hospice. I didn't want to leave a minute too early, but I was called in and I am being called out. It has been very intense, and very valuable. God bless you.

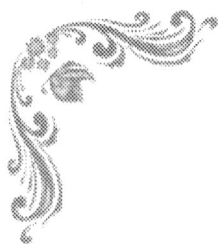

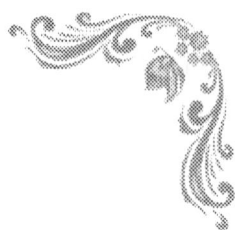

Chapter Three

IS LAUGHTER PART
OF DYING?

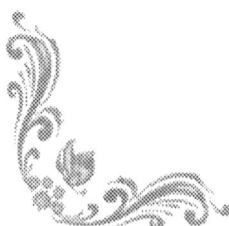

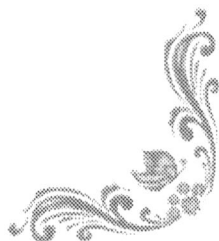

JIM AND BARBIE—HE AIN'T HEAVY...

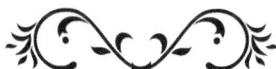

*J*need to tell you about Jim and his wife Barbie. I had received Report[5] on these folks, and they were both still working. Jim was the patient. He was diagnosed with lung cancer and there was nothing more the doctors could do. He was 51 years old and worked in construction. Barbie worked with him.

Usually I see people the day after they are assessed, but it was hard to track these people down. I had talked to Barbie on the phone a few times and found she was easy to talk to. She just laughed at EVERY-THING. She was an amazing woman. They were always busy and I was trying to find a way to get to see them. Finally I said, "Well, you all have to stop long enough to eat lunch, right? Let's meet for lunch." So I met them at the Famous Amos.

That first day I looked at this man and thought he had the bright-est, bluest eyes I had ever seen. He and Barbie were so down to earth and laughing with the joy of life. Jim said he wanted to work as long as possible. They lived in a little trailer (they had an RV), and they had a 14-year-old son, Bryan, who was being home schooled.

I started making appointments to see them in their environment. They did have a house they visited occasionally, about an hour and a half away from the city. Week after week I would go see Jim and

Barbie wherever their construction jobs happened to be, making sure he had sufficient pain medication and his symptoms were controlled.

One day, I got a call saying that Jim had passed out at the construction site. As I was talking to Barbie on the phone, the crew moved him safely into a lawn chair. That's when Barbie knew that the people who worked with Jim were aware of his illness, and how much they loved Jim. So Jim just sat in a lawn chair and continued to supervise and run the business. Barbie just laughed and carried on.

As time went on, I started meeting him at the trailer. By this time he couldn't go to work, he was so weak. This man was about 6' 2", and he had started to lose weight very rapidly. He wanted to know what death would be like, so we would talk about it.

One time we talked for about two hours. He told me about when he was "saved." He said he had been a miserable kind of man—a "bar room brawl" kind of person—and then he and Barbie started building an addition on to this church. The pastor of the church had invited them to come to church services and started talking to them about spiritual things.

Years ago, Jim had heard about God, about His saving grace and about what God could do for him, but he didn't really ever do anything about it. Jim said that one day, as he was sitting in the back of the church, he just went forward and accepted what the preacher was telling him. He said it CHANGED his life. Three months later he was diagnosed with terminal cancer. He said it was perfect timing.

He felt bad about not doing more for other people throughout his life. But I assured him that he WAS doing a lot now. Just hearing his story was like going to church for me.

Jim's illness progressed. Barbie, a little five-foot feisty woman, was out working their construction business because Jim was unable to work. I visited him regularly, and we would both sit in captain's chairs in the RV, talking.

When Barbie came home, I would talk to her about how she was going to support herself. She had started going to phlebotomy school at night and was working construction during the day. These people had a HARD life.

You meet all kinds of people in Hospice, and Jim and Barbie really impressed me. No matter what, they always had a smile. They were always concerned about the other person. They were excellent role models on "how to be"—on "how to live." Barbie always laughed and had a cheerful spirit.

One day Barbie was in her van when a car hit her, and she came home with her neck in a brace. She had chronic headaches from this car accident, yet she was still LAUGHING. Now, that's the one thing I CANNOT do when I get headaches…I cannot laugh. But Barbie could laugh about anything, anytime.

Then she got in another car accident. After that, she couldn't use her right arm. By this time, Jim was really declining and needed this little woman to help him. And she did! She never complained, no matter what. She just did it, and laughed.

I could always talk to Barbie about Jim's decline. We were very open and honest with each other about how it would happen and what she would need.

I will never forget when Jim started to hallucinate. Some people just do that. Although I'm laughing as I am telling this, it really wasn't funny, because it scared him. We reviewed his medications, but believed the medications weren't causing the hallucinations. And, anyway, we could not have cut back on any of them. So we put him on a little Haldol[6] to try to control it.

One of my main concerns is about the patients' bowels. With pain medication, bowels can really slow down and the patient can get constipated. When you can't get a patient's bowels regulated, that is very difficult for the patient. So I always want to avoid this.

One day, when I walked in, Jim said, "I'm going to make your day!"

I asked, "How are you going to do that?"

Jim and Barbie began telling me a story, each filling in parts of it: One night Jim was making a commotion in the bathroom and Barbie went to see what was happening. Seems he was in the bathroom with a big stick, and he was trying to push something down the toilet.

He said, "Barbie, Barbie, there's a animal in the toilet…there's a big animal in the toilet…a pig or something."

By this time, Barbie started laughing. She thought for sure he was hallucinating again. She walked into the bathroom and there was the BIGGEST bowel movement she had ever seen. It couldn't go down the toilet, so Jim was trying to push it down with the stick. She said that neither one of them had ever seen anything like this. It was hysterical!

Jim said it was truly as big as an animal, and he knew this would make my day. He just wanted to let me know that his bowels had actually moved. It should have gone into the *Guinness Book of World Records* as the largest human bowel movement ever! It's funny how people start joking with you about things you have to take seriously, when these are what you focus on professionally.

Anyway, it DID make my day, it truly did.

On a subsequent visit, Jim was in bed and I was talking to Barbie. She said, "Patty, he is dying. He has said goodbye to everybody. He has said goodbye to me." At that point, I knew that he would be okay. He just had this peace about him. He had those beautiful blue eyes that showed God right through them.

Jim always said he wanted to be at home when he died. So we packed him up, and he and Barbie got in the RV and went back to their house near another town. I did not see Jim again. But I kept in touch with Barbie by cell phone. Jim wanted to go to their church one more time to see all of his friends, so they did.

Barbie told me later how peaceful Jim's death was. He had looked at her and said, "Thank you for being such a good wife. Thank you, thank you." Then he turned over and stopped breathing. Barbie had taken care of everything. As she told me this story, in between her crying, she was laughing. I loved that about Barbie.

We had a memorial service for Jim at the Hospice Center in our little chapel, during which his family invited me to stand up and talk about Jim. So I told this story: They say you can tell a hospice nurse, because their wardrobe consists of black and off-black. I do love to wear black. Anyway, I guess I had shown up several weeks in a row wearing black. So one day Jim said, "You know...I've noticed that you keep wearing black...are you trying to tell me that I'm dying?"

I thought that was the funniest thing. So, for the memorial service, I wore the brightest colors I could find, to represent that his spirit was ALIVE. Jim would have appreciated that.

After the memorial service was over and everyone else had left, Barbie and I were standing in the chapel. She had the urn with Jim's ashes. She said, "You know, I haven't actually gotten a good look at Jim."

I said, "What?"

She said, "I haven't really looked at his ashes."

So, we unscrewed the top of his urn, and…my gosh, he was a big guy. The urn was HEAVY. I never realized that when someone is cremated, that the ashes can be so heavy. But I guess a 200-pound man, even when you get him down to pure ash, still carries some weight! We thought about the song "He Ain't Heavy, He's My Brother" at the same time, and started laughing. I guess you had to be there.

I talked to Barbie later, and it just seems that sometimes bad things happen to good people. When she and Bryan drove back to their house later that day, they saw that the house had burned down. Apparently lightning had hit their house and burned it to the ground. The only things that they salvaged from the house were some pictures, Bryan's guitar, and a couple of little relics. But their house and everything else was gone.

As Barbie told me this, she laughed. She said, "You know, what else can happen here? There is just nothing else that can happen."

She taught me something…that you can always laugh. No matter what happens in life…you can always laugh, even if you are going through hell. You can laugh and somehow get through it.

MY GOLFER

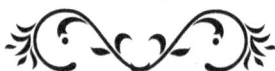

I met Mr. Shock one morning at his home. I was told on Report that he was a golfer and I knew we would relate because I also play golf. I am a VERY poor golfer. But I understand the obsession and the personality. So I was anxious to meet this person.

I went to his house and, sure enough, not being able to play golf was the thing that upset him most about having lung cancer. He was part of an asbestosis case with the armed forces and was oxygen-dependent when I first met him. He could go outside for short periods of time, but he couldn't play golf at all. He had been an obsessive golfer.

First I let him know that I understood. I got him set up in the walker so he could lean forward and putt, and if he did fall forward, I showed him how to lean against the walker. I also got him one of those little machines that can be used indoors, where you hit the ball and it returns it to you, if you do it right.

Well, on my next visit, before I could assess him, he decided to "test the nurse." I could assess him if I got a hole-in-one. God was with me that day—I hit the hole in one and was "allowed" to assess him.

This started a series of "Let's see if we can get Patty!" This man had a very dry sense of humor. His name was "Chaarlie," from "New

Yaark," along with "Maarjorie" his wife, and his daughters, Laurie, Amanda, and Karen. Laurie was the main person there with him most of the time.

So I just became part of their family. Every time I would go to the house, they would have something crazy planned for me. It was the funniest thing. Each visit he would graciously allow me to take his blood pressure and listen to his lungs. I couldn't hear a thing in his lungs, but he was in good pain control.

The next visit, he gave me this little hole-in-one toy for my desk. It had "hole-in-one" imprinted on the top: You lifted it up and, sure enough, there was a ball in the hole. It was very cool.

The family found out that I am a vegetarian, which they thought was absolutely hysterical. So on another occasion they gave me a little box that said, "3-piece chicken dinner." You opened it up, and it had three kernels of corn in it!

Mr. Shock did not like to be pushed around in the wheelchair, but at the same time his physical limitations made it difficult for him to get around with the walker. His symptoms were mainly shortness of breath, so we got some Ativan[7] for him and he started taking those with him when he would go out for short visits.

One day, I decided it was my turn to play a prank. He had this little dog named Winston, so one day I took this pile of fake doggie poop—a big old rubber pile. Now, Winston is a little, teeny terrier—really tiny. He fits into two hands. Well, I put this fake doggie poop down on the floor, and said "Oh. Oh. Oh, my gosh."

Mr. Shock looked down, and he said "Wi-i-inston!"

It was then that I realized that you don't pull this kind of joke on someone who gets short of breath easily. He went so crazy over Winston making this big pile on the floor that his anxiety level rose and he became very short of breath. I decided to keep my pranks to myself next time. Because his joy was basically "getting Patty's goat" and that was okay with me.

Laurie and Amanda told me that they wanted to do something nice for me when I came the following week. They said they wanted to wash my car while I was visiting with their dad. I thought that was really sweet.

The next visit I was orienting another nurse, so she was riding with me. As I pulled in the driveway, there were Laurie and Amanda in camouflage green combat outfits. They started throwing water balloons at my windshield! Honestly! They must have had a hundred of those water balloons!

The nurse and I were in the car and I had not thought to mention anything to her about the car wash. She was saying, "Oh my gosh! Oh my gosh!" I just turned on the windshield wipers and laughed and laughed—told her not to sweat it. Laurie and Amanda in their combat gear throwing water balloons—THAT was my car wash!

Another day I walked in the house and Amanda was dressed up in a nurse's outfit. She had on this nurse's hat, along with a horrible blond wig, and a stethoscope around her neck. She put on this act as if she were me. She began mimicking me, saying "What is your blood pressure today?" And, "Mr. Shock, have your bowels moved? You know, it is very important. We must move, move, move! Or we stop, stop, stop, stop! Which is it? Which is it?" She went on and on. I had never seen myself characterized in person before. It was just hysterical!

The next week when I went to see Mr. Shock, I was orienting a physician from a local hospital. I just could not resist—I asked him if he would help me play a prank on Mr. Shock. Fortunately, he had a good sense of humor and agreed to my plan.

Mr. Shock had shingles on the lower part of his body, which was very painful but clearing up. I had not seen much of a rash or any other evidence of the disease on my previous visit, but he told me on the phone that Monday morning that he had this very weird rash that was coming around his back. By this time, the man knew that he was dying, and with the relationship we had built, I felt like I could really joke with him about pretty much anything—as long as it didn't get him short of breath.

So this physician and I went to the house for a visit. I was assessing Mr. Shock and we were all very serious. Marjorie, his wife, was there and two of his daughters.

I looked at the rash and said, "You know, I'm really just a nurse and my experience in assessing rashes is very limited. Doctor, would you assess this and give us your opinion on it? I mean, since you're here and everything."

So, he put gloves on, and he walked around to look at Mr. Shock's back. He said, "Hmm, hmm! Hmm, hmm!"

Mr. Shock was asking, "What? What is it?" He was starting to get a little bit anxious.

The physician said, "Does it hurt here?"

Mr. Shock said, "No."

"Does it hurt here?"

"No," said Mr. Shock.

"Does it itch?"

"Well, just a little bit at night."

"Ohooo!" said the doctor.

"WHAT?"

The physician leaned back, took his gloves off—snapping them for effect—and asked, "Can I put these somewhere where they won't get anything contaminated?"

Margaret said, "Oh yes," and she brought out a special garbage bag just for the gloves.

He put them in the bag and said, "Just let me wash my hands."

He washed his hands and came back to where we were sitting. He said, "Mr. Shock, I have to tell you that you have contracted the disease Chinese Belly Rot."

For a moment Mr. Shock's eyes got big and he looked at me.

Laurie, Amanda, and Marjorie started laughing hysterically. The look on Mr. Shock's face was enough. I said, "I gotcha! I gotcha good! You've got Chinese Belly Rot, bud!" We all got such a good laugh.

Around Christmas time Mr. Shock began getting very weak. He was having a hard time getting out of bed in the morning. I was there the morning of Christmas Eve, and he said, "I want to see you and your daughter on Christmas Eve."

I thought that was so sweet. So I took my 13-year-old daughter to meet him that evening. He didn't know her, but he gave her a Tweety Bird watch, not even knowing that Tweety Bird was one of her favorites. He gave me a beautiful little crystal candle. I got to see his daughters all dressed up and the house was beautifully decorated. It was a lovely time—a bittersweet time for me, as I knew his time was short.

He wanted to make it through Christmas, and then he just wanted to make it to New Year's Eve. I went to the house New Year's Eve and he was quietly lying in bed. He was definitely declining. It was such a strange thing to see him that way after all we had been through together.

I sat with him and he said, "Patty, I am so weak. What do I do? What's the next step?"

I told him, "You can't do things alone anymore. It's not safe. Call someone to help you to the bedside commode when you need it. You will at some point go into a coma state. You won't know what's going on, and you will basically just go to sleep."

He said, "Okay." He looked at me a moment. Then he said, "I have just enjoyed this time with you. You've become one of my girls."

I loved this man and his family and it was so difficult to let him go.

That was near the weekend. On Monday I had gotten the Report that Mr. Shock had died. He had gotten up from the bedside commode. He had looked at his wife and said, "Marjorie, I love you." He had told all the girls to take care of their mother and, in his own brash way, he had told them that he loved them too. Then he just lay down and died so peacefully.

Next Christmas, the girls came to see me. Laurie had made me a "sister" pillow. She had made one for each of her sisters and one for me as an honorary member of the family, because I was "one of the girls."

Laurie later told me that the last six months of her father's life (the time when I was with him) were the happiest times because he had somebody to play pranks on—me. What a doll! He would always say that the girls wanted him to do something, like it was never his idea.

About a year later I was walking through a store and all of a sudden I heard, "Patty. There's Patty." I turned around and there was Laurie. She started talking about things they had done with Marjorie, and I said, "What about Marjorie?"

She looked at me, her eyes watering, and she said, "You didn't know?" She said, "Mom had done all the funeral planning and everything, and then she died a month later." She had gotten ill, gone to the hospital, and died.

So Laurie and I stood there in the store, crying. She told me all about it. It was like my own mother had died. This family was very much a part of me.

A few months passed and a quilt showed up at Hospice. It was a quilt that the girls had donated. It hangs on the wall at the Center for Caring in the Inpatient Hospice Unit. It is beautiful, and every time I pass by there, I think of this family and how much they mean to me.

I saw Laurie again in the same store and told her about writing this book. I told her how I would share with other people her family's experiences.

She said, "Oh, Dad would love for you to do that!"

It was so weird, because I felt his spirit right there with us. It was so very real to both of us. He was my golfer and my friend, and I will never forget him.

MR. LANE

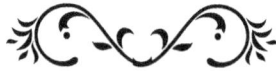

*W*hen I first met my patient Mr. Lane, he was in a state of
denial. I took his blood pressure and joked around with
him a little bit. He was still up and about and would
joke back. His wife's name was Lois—a darling. She just wanted to
make him happy. They had a beautiful little country house. I met his
daughters and his son, and they were about my age. They just loved
their daddy.

As I visited over the weeks, I built a relationship with him. If he had
a symptom, I would call and tell the doctor about it. Sometimes I
would prefer talking to the P.A.[8], because she was more responsive. We
changed his medications a little bit, and I taught the family about the
changes.

Then his appetite started decreasing. Families and caretakers have
the hardest time when patients stop wanting to eat, because food is
"love" in our culture. They think that people get better when you feed
them—"Let me feed you and make you feel better." He stopped wanting to eat, and that was a big deal for his family. What they didn't realize is that when people stop eating, that's how God prepares us to leave
our body. It is a natural reaction. When you stop eating and you go
into a fasting state, the "feel good" hormones start being injected into
your body naturally.

But I have seen people shove food down their loved one's throat when the person can't swallow. The mechanism of swallowing starts shutting down and at the same time the decrease of appetite happens. If you feed a person who can't swallow, it gives them a choking sensation, and that's really not good. People just don't want to eat when their body is shutting down. I compare it to the summertime, when you may just not feel like eating.

Over a period of time, Mr. Lane started spending more time in his room. I convinced his family that they really needed a hospital bed. He had a recliner next to the bed and he would get in that chair and sit for hours. I would have long conversations with his daughters. The whole time I was treating their father the way I would have wanted my dad to be treated. They were so sweet. Mrs. Lane would go from denial and disbelief, to reality and understanding. Sometimes I would leave the Lane house crying, realizing what they must be going through.

Then the family brought in a home health aide to help with bathing and hygiene. That was a big deal, because Mr. Lane didn't want anybody to look at him. He was very, very conservative—very shy. He never would let anybody but his wife see him, and she said that she had scarcely seen him throughout their entire marriage.

Eventually he became recliner-bound. Then he could not hold back his urine, and their nights became very long. I think that is very hard on families—being up all night, the patient getting restless. Of course, we got him some medication for restlessness and calmed him down.

There were a few good nights. But he started getting agitated and trying to get up in the middle of the night, and they would try to calm him down. He was trying to climb over the side-rails. This is another problem—when the family doesn't want to sedate their loved one. I think they are afraid they are going to somehow hasten his death.

The family starts to get exhausted. I think it is part of the process. They become so exhausted that they HAVE to start letting go. They have to start seeing how it would be so much better for that person, and for them, if they just accepted the fact that the person is going to leave. But this is hard. This is very, very hard for everyone.

People sometimes become very reliant on the Hospice team. If you have a good social worker, you can share the burdens. But most of the responsibility, I have noticed, falls on the nurse, if she has compassion. This is where you either begin to distance yourself or become very enmeshed in the family issues. You start leaving more houses crying, when you dread going to the home because you don't know whether the patient is going to have a good day or a bad day. You start rejoicing when the patient can actually talk to you.

On this particular day Mr. Lane had started filling up with fluid. What bothers me the most in the dying process is the gurgling. They call it the "death rattle," and I really hate that sound. This man was full of fluid, so that was my priority.

I said to him, "Mr. Lane, can I please put in a Foley catheter?[9] It will make it easier on your family." Sometimes you have to convince these patients, especially the men, that putting in a Foley catheter or doing some other health measure will be easier on their families. A lot of men in that generation—those in their 70's—are more concerned about the care and comfort of their family than they are about themselves. He did allow me to put in a Foley catheter and he stopped sounding quite so "wet," and that was good.

I also ordered a scopolamine patch. This patch was once used—and probably still is—for seasickness. People put it behind their ear on their neck so they wouldn't get seasick. We use it in Hospice for drying up secretions—the secretions that just naturally occur sometimes in the lungs.

This gurgling is a most disturbing sound. As soon as I hear it begin, I start working to make it go away, because it really bothers me. I guess it's my sense of hearing, because it doesn't seem to bother the patient. Sometimes they can be talking and gurgling away, and they don't even notice it. But the families do, and they start thinking, "Oh, my gosh, he is going to drown."

I started Mr. Lane on a "scop patch" and put him on Benadryl. Our standing orders were "1 to 2 Benadryl q. 6-8h. p.r.n."[10] I put him on Benadryl every six hours around the clock, and they gave it to him rectally. In order to convince them to do this, I explained to them that it would help the sound go away.

So now you get the picture—I was trying to dry him up. He was in bed. He had entered the dying process.

I went to the house the next day. The family had had a bad night. They were up with him, and he was restless. He was talking to people that they couldn't see, which is very common in people who are dying. Usually they are talking to deceased people. They start talking to their mom or dad or Aunt Lucille or Uncle Harvey or whatever deceased people were in their family. I truly believe that they are communicating with the other side; they are between this world and the next. Sometimes they get this look on their face that they are not really here and they are not really there. It's the most profound experience to see a person "sitting on the fence" about whether to stay or whether to go. But it is a very difficult time for the family. This is when I encourage family members to say what they need to say. Tell the person it's okay to go, but also give that person some time alone.

The next day the family called me at 8:29 AM. I went over not knowing what I was going to find. The daughter said they had had another bad night. Mr. Lane was lying in the recliner with his eyes rolled back. He was very restless, very agitated, and he sounded like he was under water. I could hear him gurgling the minute I walked in the door, and I thought, oh, my God. I was just praying, "God help me, God help me, God help me." I just kept thinking, if this were my dad... I believe that is the number one thing that has made me a good Hospice nurse—but it is also what made me feel panic in this situation. So I made sure that, when I walked in, I maintained a calm composure.

Mr. Lane's family was very insistent on getting him back to bed. This man was dying, and these folks did not want to leave him in the chair. Some people just LIKE to be in their recliners. There is nothing wrong with that, but Mr. Lane's family didn't want to hear about that. So I got him back into bed.

Then he got some clarity, looked straight at me, and tried to speak through all of this gurgling sound. It was horrible. I put on my gloves and told his daughter to get me some Benadryl, some K-Y, and some Lasix[11]. I put another patch on him. I called the pharmacy, in the meantime, and got orders for all these things. I gave him Lasix to drain

41

the fluid. I gave him Benadryl to dry him out. I gave him another patch, and waited and prayed—and waited and prayed.

Next, he insisted on standing up. He wanted to put his shorts on or something. Now, I am the last person in the world to not give someone his dying wish. So I got this man up—who is 6 feet tall. He wasn't an obese man at all, but he was heavy. Anyway, I got him to stand up. The daughters put his boxer shorts over his Foley catheter, and we were laughing already. His wife got behind him, so he wouldn't fall. It was getting hysterical.

So I was in front of him. Lois was behind him. His daughter Diane was to my left. Then his other daughter walked into the room. I had started to gently sit him down, when suddenly he fell back on top of Lois. I fell on top of him. Diane fell on top of me. The other daughter just stood there laughing at us, and this man just kept gurgling away.

It is not really funny, but it seemed so at the time. We were all laughing. He looked at us, fully lucid for a moment. Smiling and gurgling, he said, "What a way to go!" And, oh, I have never laughed so hard. I just lay on top of him and I laughed—I couldn't move because Diane was on top of me, also laughing. Well, we finally got Lois out from underneath all of us and we got Mr. Lane situated in bed, but it was truly a profound moment. A man came back from almost the "other side" to tell us that we had brought him a bit of laughter.

That was definitely memorable: the laughter, finally getting him back into bed with his shorts on, and seeing that, after all my efforts, his gurgling really was not much better. But at least he was in bed, his side-rails were up, and he was safe. That was all I could do for them at that moment.

I went into the kitchen and sobbed at the kitchen counter where I had talked to the doctor a million times before, refilled Mr. Lane's medications, or changed his medications to keep him more comfortable. And I sobbed because I knew this was the end. There was nothing more that I could do.

That's when I realized that these people had given me more than I could ever give them.

You know, to be a Hospice nurse and to be part of people's lives is basically "tucking them in"—getting them ready to go to heaven. What an honor! Sometimes I'm just in awe of the fact that God gave me this opportunity. When I see my families in the stores and around town, there is an immediate connection. We have been together through a deep and profound time in their lives, and I feel deeply honored.

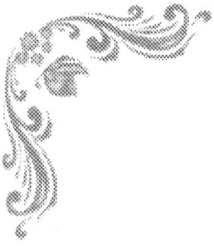

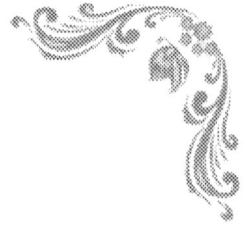

Chapter Four

LEARNING FROM
DIFFICULT SITUATIONS

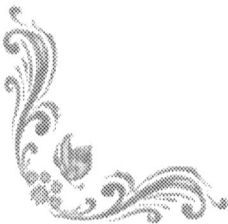

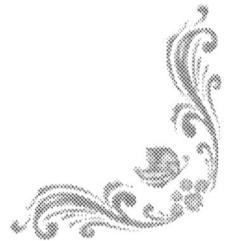

DOCUMENTATION IS IMPORTANT

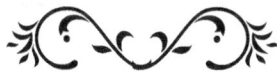

*A*lthough I hesitated to tell you about this experience, I feel a great deal of responsibility to Hospice nurses, to prepare them for some of the things that they may encounter. A lot of the stories you have read so far may have been profound, enlightening or funny, but sometimes things take a different turn. This is a story that needs to be told.

The names are different, of course, and the situation has been modified just a bit. When you work in the medical field, people can come back years later, to criticize you and your charting or procedures—for what happened—for what didn't happen—whatever. It's always a good idea to have liability insurance and to document everything carefully. People can become very angry when they are grieving, and sometimes whoever is around becomes their target.

I had a patient named Alice. Alice was this darling little lady. She was living in the home of her son and daughter-in-law. I got to the house about 4:30 one afternoon, and immediately I felt the anxiety in the atmosphere—you could have cut it with a knife. The patient was just as sweet and kind as she could be. Her most imminent problem was that she hadn't had a bowel movement in 10 days. Everybody was concerned, pushing Haley's MO, trying to get her to have a bowel movement.

I asked her, "Have you ever had an enema?"

She said, "I've had enemas my whole life."

I said, "Would you like to have one now?" And she gave birth to a baseball, and felt MUCH better. And that "baseball" is, of course, figurative for a LARGE bowel movement. It could just make my whole day.

During the visit, Minerva (the daughter-in-law) was acting very agitated, asking a lot of questions. She kept coming in and out of the room where I was with the patient. She was concerned about the equipment being changed out, who to talk to, on and on. It was just hellacious. She and her husband were also trying to tell me about some medical information that they read on-line, was I aware of it, and shouldn't I be doing something like that? They seemed to question my intelligence and expertise. I was tired and just wanted to care for my patient.

I made every effort to answer their questions and remain calm, and yet take care of my patient—which was my primary concern.

Two days later I went back for a second visit. They had hired a caregiver who came to the house every afternoon. They would tell her everything she needed to do and she was competent at doing whatever was required. I felt very comfortable with the patient's care.

Throughout my time with this patient, I would call Minerva often. She would be frantic, asking me questions about things I had already explained. I would explain again, and then she would seem fine.

Alice had some skin breakdown on her buttocks. We had put a duoderm[12] on her buttocks, and there was apparently a misunderstanding about its usage. I had said to leave it on as long as possible, for at least three days.

I sent over one of the triage nurses, because Minerva still didn't understand. But she continued to call in, saying, "I don't understand about the duoderm."

When the duoderm is applied to the backside, it's hard to keep it clean. When you are wiping, you don't want to get feces underneath.

Sometimes the duoderm comes off, and that's what the caregiver was doing. She was taking it off for cleaning purposes.

On one occasion Minerva said, "Am I EVER going to see a nurse?" (This was when I had just been there two days prior.)

I said, "Of course, but you're working during the day. I can send someone out for you when you get home from work, if you would like."

She said, "That won't be necessary."

I said, "Well, you want to see an RN, so let me send someone out after eight o'clock."

So, at eight o'clock that next night, Hospice sent a triage nurse to the house, to show Minerva how to apply the duoderm. I hoped this would help to settle Minerva down.

The triage nurse saw me next day in my office and said that this family really had it out for me. They told her that they had not seen an RN in two weeks.

I could not believe it. I had spent more time at this house than I had my own house!

They had told her, "Patty has problems of her own."

It really bothered me that they doubted my integrity. They also said that I didn't know what I was doing, and that I never checked her bowels. Well, I had spent more time on this lady's bowels than on anything else, because that is such a crucial thing. Your bowels control your whole well-being. Minerva's Report to this triage nurse really made me angry.

I called the home and talked to the patient's son. Unfortunately, I didn't have enough sense to talk it out with my supervisor first, to diffuse my own anger, frustration, and disbelief.

When I talked to the son, I said, "I just heard that Minerva said that I hadn't been there in two weeks, and that I hadn't been checking your mother's bowels. I really don't appreciate having my nursing integrity questioned, because I am one of the best Hospice nurses that you will encounter. I was there on Monday. Minerva was there for an hour of that visit, and then she left for work. But I saw her on Monday. Also

I want to assure you that I have checked your mother's bowels every single time that I've been there, and we've been keeping track of it. Minerva said that the caregiver was also doing enemas every day to disimpact her."

He said he didn't know that. Then he talked about how the aide said that when the duoderm came off it was just ripping her skin off, and it was heartbreaking for them.

I said, "The aides aren't supposed to be taking that duoderm OFF. It is supposed to stay ON. I have gone over this with them numerous times."

It was definitely a "no win" situation. After I hung up, I questioned if I should have called at all.

At this point, I started calling Minerva at work at the end of every single visit. I also documented each visit carefully, because I had a sense that these folks could be dangerous for a medical person coming into the home. They had such misdirected anger.

As Alice declined, the situation became very distorted. I was working in Triage on a Saturday before a holiday, and Minerva had called Triage asking, "Where's the nurse?"

Alice was supposed to be checked every four days for impaction, and I had scheduled a visit for her for the following Monday, a holiday. This was written up on her chart. But Minerva was angry. She said, "You all aren't doing ANYTHING. We haven't seen a nurse. We don't know what is going on!"

Thank heavens it was my supervisor that answered the phone. She said, "Well, I have it written down right here that Patty was out there on Friday and checked your Mom for impaction."

Minerva was cursing and making accusations about me, inferring I was not taking care of the patient. She was so hostile.

My supervisor said, "You know, I don't appreciate that kind of language."

That just set Minerva off even more. She just started ranting and raving.

The supervisor said that she would not tolerate that kind of language from this lady. She said she would send someone on Monday because that would be the fourth day, and that my documentation was accurate and everything appeared to be in order.

As I was listening to this phone call, I was remembering that just the day before I had worked extensively with Brantley and Minerva. I had suggested that they at least come look at the Hospice Center, just in case it got too much to handle at home.

They did come to the Hospice Center and I showed them the facility. While they were there, I ordered some moisture barrier cream for Alice's behind and a new medication for her mouth. I suggested that they pick it up at the pharmacy while they were there, so they could have it right away. They were leaving the Hospice Center at four o'clock and I assumed, since they were so concerned about Alice's comfort, that they would take it right home to be used immediately.

I wanted to follow up, just to be thorough, so I called them at eight o'clock that night. They were just getting home. Minerva said, "Oh yeah, we picked up the moisture barrier ointment, and we got the mouth medication."

I said, "Well, have you applied it?"

She said, "No, we just got home."

I was shocked. I said, "Well, Brantley was so concerned about Alice's buttocks and his mom's comfort that I wanted to be sure you got that medication as soon as possible. Our couriers usually don't get there until 8:30 or 9:00 P.M., and you were so upset about that last time, that I wanted to make it more convenient."

I said this to make sure that my intentions were clarified.

She said, "Oh no. We just got home and everything is fine."

Later I heard that she had called, saying that I MADE them pick up the medications at The Hospice Center instead of having it couriered out.

This just shows that you can have the best of intentions as a nurse. However, people who are experiencing the loss of a loved one sometimes need to place blame. As a medical professional, especially a

Hospice person who represents the fact that their family member is going to die, YOU sometimes become the target.

As a result of this, I went back through my documentation in detail and made sure my notes were clear. I documented every single day that I had called Minerva. I documented all of my visits. I documented all of my phone calls. I documented, documented, documented.

I didn't know how the grieving process was going to be for them. However, I did know that there was a large element of persecution with this, and I was the target. You should ALWAYS document very well, no matter what the situation, because we deal with life and death.

This gives new meaning to the prayer, "God, grant me the serenity to accept the things I cannot change, the courage to change the things I can, and the wisdom to know the difference." All I could control was my documentation and the care I gave the patient, and I could pray for these people.

I put this story into this book because this is a reaction that you may run into, and I want you to be prepared. I want to validate your frustration at being unable to change some situations. It's not always about going out there and feeling good, feeling like you're completing a mission. Just be secure in the fact that you do the very best you can.

MR. SOCRATES

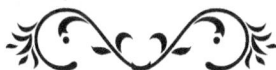

his next story is traumatic. However, I consider it an honor to be able to go into people's homes, visit them personally, and meet the greatest minds on the planet. And it is a story that deserves to be included.

I had this patient who did not feel he needed Hospice to come in. But, my dad is a real intellectual and so is my mom, so I tried to relate to him on that level. I said, "Okay, I understand you don't want Hospice in. What about special visits from a person who just wants to pick your brains?" I always did whatever it took, because I really don't know how I would feel about Hospice coming into my house if I didn't know anything about it.

I enjoyed talking to this man—he was brilliant. He was a writer and had also practiced law. I would visit him and pick his brain for nuggets of knowledge, and also practice good symptom control. We also went on the "joke of the week" program, where he would tell me a joke and I would tell him a joke. We had a great time. I'll call him Mr. Socrates.

The man had no pain at all, but he was as orange as a pumpkin. His liver was definitely affected. He had pancreatic cancer, and someone had told him that pancreatic cancer was very painful.

His physician was very responsive—I would call her whenever I had a problem. We got Mr. Socrates on Ecotrin[13], because he had started having some aches and pains. I wanted to be sure he was in no pain, because of a previous experience he had taking care of his wife some years before. She had cancer also, and had died a very painful and horrible death. She was not in the Hospice program, but in the hospital. She was given massive doses of morphine. He later told me that she had metastasis to the bone. Morphine is good for most cancer pain, but specifically for bone pain it is not the drug of choice—there are other things. So he had this prior situation in his head.

I had our social worker on the case who frequently visited the house. This man wanted all of his paperwork done perfectly. His will was in order. His DNR[14] was in order—everything. I really respected this person for taking care of all of these things appropriately.

It was Friday afternoon when Mr. Socrates called me, something he had never done before. He asked if he could get a hospital bed, because he was getting so weak. He said he just thought it would be more comfortable if he could lift his head.

I said, "Sure, and I'd like to come visit you."

He said, "No that's not necessary—I just want to be more comfortable, and I'm ready for a bed." I knew as our visits had continued that he was becoming more accepting of his diagnosis. He always said everything was "fine."

The weekend came and went. Monday morning I got a call from his daughter, saying the home health aide had found him. During a thunderstorm he had gone into the bathroom and shot himself.

This story is in the book because although this kind of situation occurred, none of the warning signs were there. I think I would have seen them. A highly skilled social worker would have seen any symptoms, had these been present. We have Risk Assessments written up by our social workers when they see the signs, but none was written up on him. The doctor didn't see it either—she was amazed when she found out.

The daughter said to me, "My dad is the cruelest man in the whole world. I can't believe he would do that to us." What he did was leave his daughter, a beautiful granddaughter who was about seven years old, and the home health aide that found him, with that memory. He was afraid of dying in pain, but nobody knew to what extent. No one suspected suicide.

For a time after that happened, I went into a depression of sorts. Because of my role in Hospice, in order to be effective I did have to get somewhat involved. I did have to relate. One can be a decent nurse and just go in and be completely detached, but I cannot do it and maybe that was my downfall. Maybe this is why I'm at a burnout state right now, because I got too involved. But it has been a good six years.

The people at Hospice comforted me during this time. Hospice has programs available for people to talk to professionals about people in a serious situation.

Sad things happen and sometimes no matter what you do, it is not a good death. If someone had shared a similar experience with me as a Hospice nurse, I believe I would have had a faster healing process.

I did live through it, and I wasn't responsible for it. But I will never forget it.

MY LITTLE BOSNIAN

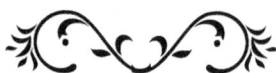

’m going to tell you about someone else who affected my life PRETTY heavily—in a whole different way. I got Report that this patient didn’t want to see ANY nurses. Well, maybe one nurse would be okay, especially if she were blond. Nobody living in this house spoke English. They all spoke Bosnian. They said the patient spoke some English, but not very much. I love a challenge, so I prayed about it. I decided to go, fully realizing I might be thrown out.

When I got to the home I saw several little kids outside, and a woman answered the door. She was very pleasant. I looked in her eyes and saw that she was very tired. She didn’t speak English, so she just took me in to see the patient.

He was paralyzed from the waist down and had very advanced cancer. He lay in bed with a trapeze handle overhead for lifting himself. He couldn’t look at me at first, so I said, “Ollie? Am I saying your name correctly? Is it Ollie?”

Then he turned and looked at me, and said, “Yes, that is my name.”

And I said, “Ollie, I’m planning on being your nurse. I am not going to bother you. I’m just going to come see you, and you can call me whenever you need to.” I set up a plan for him and I asked, “Do you understand what I’m saying to you?”

He nodded.

I said, "Ollie, is it okay if I take your blood pressure?"

He said, "Yes," and held his arm up.

It was kind of a stilted little conversation there for a while, but I asked him some questions to build rapport and to be sure he understood me. I said, "Can you teach me some Bosnian, so that I can communicate with your family?"

So Ollie taught me how to say "pain" and "goodbye" and "hello" in Bosnian. Now that the situation is over, all I can remember is *doe vea jay nya*[15], which means goodbye. But somehow we were able to communicate.

That day, I was having a particularly down day. I was low on faith. I looked at him, I sat down, and we connected eye-to-eye. He had these coal-black eyes. And I said, "Ollie, how are you inside? How are you doing spiritually?" I don't know why I asked that question. It just seemed right at the time.

He looked up at the ceiling and said, "I'm just here. This is what God has planned. All I can do is give glory to God for the time that I have, which is just right now. That is all we ever have—right now."

As he was saying this, a child (about 18 months old) came in and looked at his grandfather. Ollie just kind of smiled at the child and there was pure love in his eyes.

I asked, "Ollie, are you going to let me come back?"

And he said, "Only YOU."

"Okay," I said. "If I get hit by a bus, it will have to be somebody else. But as long as I can, it will be me."

And he said, "Okay."

So I left him and walked back through the house. Trying to practice my Bosnian, I said, "Doe vea jay nya" to his wife, and I thought she was going to jump out of her skin with joy.

I also saw another little Bosnian woman with a draped head working around the house—that woman was Ollie's mother. Ollie had a daughter-in-law who could speak some English, but she did not live there. I talked to her quite a bit, especially at first when Ollie had pain. But as time went on, he and I learned to communicate pretty well. I started to look forward to the visits, and he seemed to tolerate me.

I will never forget the day I tried to talk him into letting me use a Foley catheter. I explained it to him, and that is when his English started to falter. He started speaking Bosnian to me. I found out that he also knew some Spanish. It was really funny, because his Bosnian was decreasing, but he could remember Spanish. So we spoke Spanish to each other, and I thought—this is a God thing; it has to be.

My Spanish was much worse than his, but I did have a Spanish dictionary that I took to the house. I didn't have a Bosnian dictionary. Hospice tried to get a translator for me, but the translator did not become available until after Ollie died. So I guess we didn't need one after all. I have learned that LOVE is a universal language. I knew that the God in Ollie loved me, and I knew that the God in me could love his family and him. And we just communicated on that level, and somehow it worked.

Ollie did allow the Foley catheter. That went okay, and then I had to explain to his wife how to empty the bag and clean up. His wife had the most gentle, sweet spirit—but Ollie could get pretty rough with her. He would get frustrated and tell her to go away. All she wanted to do was to take care of him. I taught her by showing her. Then she would do it and I would give positive reinforcement, and she understood. We communicated with love. I can't explain it any other way, because by all rights this should not have gone well.

His pain would get out of control every once in a while, and they would sometimes misunderstand the instructions. They would give him the patch AND the pills when he was supposed to stop taking the pills. Then they took the patch off AND stopped giving him the pills. It would be a matter of me catching up on Monday with the crazy things that had happened since I left, but we managed to communicate and we kept him straightened out pretty well.

As Ollie declined, he was not able to eat. Then he stopped drinking fluids as well. I sat down with his daughter-in-law (the one who spoke some English) and went over the dying process with her. I told her she needed to explain this carefully to her family. She agreed to talk to them.

One day I went to see Ollie. It was so hot in the house. I think it was because he was their sole means of support and they couldn't afford any cooling. They had only come over to the United States about three years prior, and he had been diagnosed about six months prior. That morning his sons were there, his daughter was there (whom I had not met before). She took it all in as I again went through signs and symptoms for these people. I again asked them to explain all of this to their mother and grandmother. And they agreed.

Well, that afternoon I was driving down the road and got a call on my alpha pager (which gives text messages). It said—"Please come ASAP. Social worker died. Come to Bosnian's house now."

The social worker was obviously pretty upset when she entered that message, because it was the Bosnian man who had died—not the social worker! So I called the house and talked to the social worker, Diane, who sounded very stressed.

"How far away are you?" she pleaded. "He has just died and all hell has broken loose! The son is bashing his head against the wall. His daughter keeps coming over to the bed, crying and passing out. I don't know what to do!!"

I was only about a mile away, so I said, "I will be there right away." I drove up the driveway and heard screaming coming from inside the house. I prayed, "Oh please God, be in this situation."

I have never seen anything like this before, but I do know that people in different cultures grieve very differently. What I learned is that you just have to let people grieve the way they need to grieve. You don't try to control them. You don't try to make them stop. You respect their ways and just try to keep everyone safe.

Flies were in the house by this time. Ollie's mother (the woman with the shawl on her head) was on the floor, sobbing. So I thought, well, she is not really controllable, but not in danger either.

Diane grabbed me and pulled me over to Ollie's daughter, who was stumbling over to him. She would cry, then pass out and fall to the floor. Could she be dying?

I took her blood pressure and her pulse. She was fine. I said, "She's okay. Just protect her head and keep her on the floor." I wanted to keep this girl on the floor for safety, and I needed to determine if Ollie was truly dead. I was listening to his heart.

His wife was in the other room, inconsolable. And the son was just sitting there, staring. We had made him stop banging his head against the concrete wall. I was afraid he would bash his head open and start bleeding, so we got him to sit and then gave him a job. He was to keep his sister still on the floor, so she wouldn't fall and hurt herself. But she just kept crying, "Daddy, Daddy, Daddy." Oh, my gosh, it's breaking my heart to remember this even now.

I pulled my social worker over to the bed and said, "You know, we need to destroy these medications."

She looked at me like I had lost my mind. But I told her, "They are going to grieve the way they are going to grieve. Everyone is safe for now."

As we were talking, the daughter got up, went over to Ollie's bed, and passed out again. I got the two boys. They picked her up, but I said, "Lay her on the floor—she can't fall if she's on the floor. Keep her there."

I sat on the bed with my social worker—everybody was hysterical one way or another.

Diane said, "Well, what do we do?"

"Well, the daughter is safe," I said. "The son's not bashing his head against the wall. Even though people are still screaming and crying, no one is in immediate danger. What we really need to do is destroy these medications, so that someone doesn't decide to take them."

So, while things were relatively under control, we went to destroy all the medications. By this time, my poor social worker was in shock. We were in the privacy of the bathroom, dumping all the medications in the toilet, and then I started to laugh.

Sometimes that happens to me at the worse possible moments— laughing at inappropriate times. It used to happen at funerals all the time. I would get so stressed that I would laugh, and I couldn't stop.

As a matter of fact, it happened at my dad's father's funeral. It is so embarrassing, but I guess it is just my way of coping.

So, I was laughing in the bathroom. We were destroying the medications, and Diane asked, "What do we do next?"

And I said, "Well, let's just try to give a little bit of comfort, okay?"

We went out and talked to the son about transporting his father's body to the funeral home.

But he said, "No, we are not letting the body go."

I thought—Oh, great! Okay! So we contacted somebody at the funeral home. They explained to us that in the Bosnian culture the family keeps the body a while, and to just call them when the family was ready. So Diane and I explained to the family how to call the funeral home when they were ready.

Diane did an excellent job. I was so impressed that she didn't turn in her resignation the next day. By this time I felt SO burned out—I just thought, please, Diane, don't quit.

When we got everything done and it was calm, I told Diane we needed to go back to the office. That's when I was reminded there are some things I can control and some things I cannot control as a nurse. And when you have done everything you can do, then you have to let go and let them handle the rest in their own way.

We went back to the office. My concern was no longer for the family, but for the social worker and for ME. This had been so stressful. I grabbed my supervisor and said, "We need to talk to you." And we told her the story. We downloaded. I have learned that when you experience things like this, it is VERY important for you to debrief. You have to, or you can't keep going.

Later, Diane asked me, "Can you believe this? Can you believe what we've been through?"

"No, I really can't," I said. "It is unbelievable."

She said, "And other people are calling and paging me—my other patients—but I'm not sure what to do."

I said, "Well, that's why we have to talk about it and tell our story, because we have to work through this and go on."

We called the family later. The body was still there. That was their culture and their way, and it was okay.

I learned after Ollie died that he was in Bosnia when all the bombing occurred during the war with the Serbs. That explained why he wouldn't allow any interpreters into his home, because they were all Serbs.

I also found out that Ollie had a lot of guilt. He was in construction and had left his family to find work, and that is when his family's home was bombed. One of his best friends was killed on the construction site because of the bombing. I learned what terrible things these people had lived through. I also learned that earlier in his life one of his sons had a twin that drowned, and he felt guilty about that.

These people had survived bombings and family loss. I thought of his mother, that little Bosnian lady with the hood—she was just like the pictures that I had seen on TV. These people had been through so much. They came over here, got into the business of marbling, and then Ollie was diagnosed with cancer. And he was the main support of the family.

I also learned about the "passing out" daughter. Apparently, she became pregnant while she was not married, and Ollie would have nothing to do with her baby. So he and this daughter were estranged. She never really spent any time with him. In fact, Ollie would not let her or her child into his room. He had disowned her completely. When he died, she had a major stress reaction and this was why she was passing out.

I will never forget the lessons I learned from this. When people die, God always takes care of the people that love Him. Ollie loved his God, I know he did. Most of all, LOVE is THE universal communicator.

MR. & MRS. RAILER

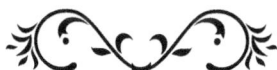

*M*any situations present themselves when you are dealing with such an intimate situation as dying. Emotions often run high. This is a difficult story about how different people deal with the dying process of those they love.

Mr. Railer, my patient, was a tall, virile guy. He was an engineer and it was through him that I learned that they actually make turbo toilets. But I need to tell you about Mrs. Railer.

Mrs. Railer was about 15 years older than Mr. Railer. My first visit was rather perfunctory. We talked, and Mr. Railer seemed to be able to verbalize very well. Mrs. Railer kept saying to me, "I need you to tell me how to do everything. I want to do it right and I don't know how to do any of this. Just tell me, and I can do it."

I assured her I would explain everything to her very carefully.

I soon realized this would be difficult. I would tell her how to do something, but never get any response from her. She would just sit there, not even nodding. She wouldn't say that she understood. Usually when people understand they give some indication with body language, eye contact, or something.

Later, Mr. Railer started getting nauseous. I called Mrs. Railer and instructed her to give him Phenergan suppositories to relieve the nausea.

I kept explaining about the suppositories, because I wanted to be sure that she understood the procedures and dosages. Finally I said to her, "Do you understand?"

She almost yelled at me over the phone, "You DON'T have to treat me like a 5-year-old! I GET IT! You are explaining this to me as if I'm stupid!"

I said, "I just need to know that YOU understand, but you are not giving me any feedback to indicate that you do understand."

Later, when I talked to the social worker, she said Mrs. Railer had told her that the next time she saw "THAT nurse" (meaning me) she was just going to punch her out for treating her like a child. So, the next time I went to the house, I had this in my mind. I took a deep breath and prayed for God to love her through me. I knew she was stressed out and I needed to know how to work with her.

She treated me fine, but she was just so persnickety. I said to her very calmly, "You know, we need to get your husband into a hospital bed, because he's a big guy and he's going to be very difficult to handle."

We had a hospital bed delivered and put in the room for Mr. Railer. No matter what we did for Mrs. Railer, nothing made her happy. She didn't like the plastic covering around it. So I took it off. She didn't like the egg crate mattress that was delivered. I said she didn't have to use it.

I was always "walking on eggshells" about how to explain things to her. She would say, "Oh, I can do this." And then she'd call back in a panic saying, "Oh, I don't know how to do anything!" This is not unusual and you cut people a lot of slack in these situations, as it is a difficult time for them.

I was standing across the bed from her when Mrs. Railer asked, "How do you TURN him?"

I was showing her how to turn him, and he was being very cooperative. I said, "Do you understand about the draw sheet?"

She slammed her hands down on the bed, and said, "You JUST keep going on and on and on explaining this!"

I looked at her calmly and said, "You know, I'm really not TRYING to be condescending toward you at all. It's just that you act like you do not understand. You look at me with this wide-eyed 'I don't get it' look, so I keep explaining it to you until I see the lights come on."

The equipment people hated to go to her house, because no matter what they brought to the house, it wasn't right. I will never forget the look on our equipment man's face as he explained his last trip. He said he took a bedside commode over there and she complained that it only had four legs! He told her it was a chair, and every chair he knew of had four legs.

So, I guess it wasn't just me—that was the good news. Anyway, God bless her heart.

I really think that sometimes people have some unexplainable dysfunction, because Mrs. Railer just did not act rationally. So I just stopped expecting her to react like a normal person, and kept explaining things to the ground, in hopes that she would listen.

She panicked at the end, even though she said she was ready. I was there one night until about five o'clock, but finally I went home, because no matter what I said, it upset her. Triage got a call that night saying that he was gurgling, and they sent a runner out. This was really good because that runner sat there with Mrs. Railer and helped her through it as Mr. Railer died.

This story is for you, Hospice workers, when you run into "damned if you do and damned if you don't" situations. Just know that all you can do is your best, and then give it to God.

MARILYN

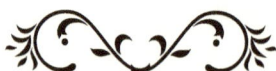

H er name was Marilyn. She was 45 years old. She had a daughter and a granddaughter, but was not much older than me. She lived in a nice little house. Her husband worked. She had cancer all through her body.

When I first met her, she was slightly orange from the metastasis to her liver. As the weeks went on, I kept thinking, "Is this lady power-loading carrots or what?!?" She was SO golden from the disease process.

Her case was very difficult medically, because every time I saw her, she was in pain. We had her on MS Contin q12[16] and were up to a dosage every eight hours. She took so much breakthrough medication, it would have sedated an average horse. But Marilyn had pain receptors all over her body that were just screaming. So every time I visited, there was a discussion with the doctor about changing her medications.

She had many friends that stayed with her. She had a hard time discussing her disease with her husband, because he was in complete denial about it. He told her things like, "You know, you CAN get well, if you just claim the healing."

Finally, I stood outside with him one day and said, "These are the facts. You're making your wife very uncomfortable, because she's got cancer. She's a Hospice patient. She knows she's dying and you're telling her it's her fault, in essence. Do you think that's making her feel more comfortable?"

When I put it in those terms, he understood and started being her advocate. We would get calls at night and on weekends about her, because her symptoms would change daily—daily! Yet she was always thinking about the other people in her life rather than herself. She was such a sweetheart.

I had never before run across what I will call spiritual abuse. This lady was a member of a very influential church. One day when I walked into her house, Marilyn was sobbing uncontrollably.

I said, "Marilyn, are you in pain? What is going on?"

When she had gathered herself together and could talk, she said, "My pastor just left. He told me that I have this cancer because I've done something bad in my past—that I brought it on myself, and that if I could just release it and claim the healing I would be well. He makes me feel like this is my fault."

She started crying again, and said, "And there's nothing I can do about it. Doesn't he know that if there was something that I could do about this, I would? I've had more laying on of hands. I've had more scripture prayed over me. I've been to healing. I eat right. I've done everything that I can do."

That's when I coined the term "spiritual abuse." I asked Marilyn if she would like to talk to our pastor. We have a Hospice chaplain who is pretty generic. She just meets people where they are. Marilyn agreed, and our chaplain went out to talk to Marilyn. I saw her the day after she had talked to our chaplain, and she looked much better. She had a peace about her that she said came from having good spiritual counsel.

Marilyn thought that if someone wanted to come see her, she was obligated to let them in and let them talk to her. That day I said to her, "Marilyn, YOUR comfort is MY job, and I don't like to do a bad job. If anybody comes in and upsets you to the point that I saw you the other day, it is in your best interest not to let that person in your home."

She looked up at me and said, "Really? I don't have to see the pastor?"

I said, "As a matter of fact, it's not in your best interest to see someone who is bringing on guilt and condemnation."

I felt a little odd saying that to her, but the effect of the kind of counsel that her pastor gave her was destructive. I can see giving that kind of counsel to someone that has a cold and "milks" it for weeks, but I couldn't see any value in this instance.

So she agreed. Marilyn did not request him to visit anymore. She only let people in who understood her situation, because she knew she was dying. She had no problem with it.

I really wasn't sure how her death was going to work out. Generally, a person will lie down, sleep more, and then go into a coma. But for some reason I just couldn't picture how hers was going to play out. There were so many people around her that loved her, and every time she moved they were in alert mode.

I came into Triage one Sunday afternoon to work. I was looking through the status sheets for my team, and I saw a mark through her page and the notation "Died."

So I started investigating. Marilyn died? What happened? I just couldn't believe it, because I had just seen her on Friday.

I was told that Marilyn got up to go take a shower. Her husband was in the living room with her child and a couple of friends. When she came out of the shower, she said, "Mark, come here. My head hurts." And then she collapsed on the floor.

He called 911 and they transported her to the hospital and intubated her. She was on life support. They ran tests and found she was fully comatose, and that she had had an aneurysm. This patient's husband, who had such a hard time with this whole process, apparently loved her enough to let her go. The family withdrew all of the life support because they knew that she didn't want to exit in that way.

I thought, "Wow! Conversations that we have with people and family members about their wishes and concerns DO make a difference!" This is exactly the way that this young woman needed to go.

God is pretty smart—really smart. Marilyn left her mark on this world. Sometimes I wish that I had known a lot of these folks before they became sick, but then I know that God's timing is always perfect in every way.

WATCH WHERE YOU SIT!

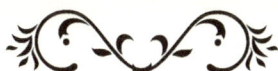

This was one of my first Hospice cases—a lesson learned early. I went to this house and when I walked in, there were cats and other various animals everywhere—just everywhere! There was this little caregiver, who was always in the kitchen. Her husband was in the back bedroom, and he sat there like a little Buddha in his chair. He was just darling. I really enjoyed them—especially him.

I can remember going through the "Signs and Symptoms of the Dying Process" with her. We sat down in the living room on the couch. As we were talking, all of a sudden I felt something seep through my pants. I didn't say anything to her because it was just so strange. We had been talking for probably an hour, when I stood up and left, and my pants WERE wet. When I got in my car, I recognized the smell as some kind of urine, which was apparently all over their furniture.

You know, people live different ways. And it really isn't any of my business how people live. But even to this day, I always touch the furniture before I sit down in anyone's house.

I guess people's priorities change when they get older, especially when they have a dying loved one in the house. But every time I left that house, I changed my clothes as soon as possible. If it was my last stop and I was going out that evening, I would take a change of clothes. I also stopped sitting down in their house.

This little man was Catholic, and he held the rosary in his hand all the time. I had a wonderful PRN nurse that worked with me on this case. She used to be one of my prayer partners. She was covering for me the last few days of his life. She was also Catholic and really helped him, because he had such a hard time letting go. She put all the right people (the priest, etc.) in contact with him. He died so peacefully. She was the right woman for the job.

And, of course, I warned her about not sitting down.

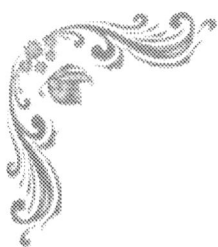

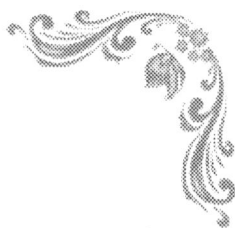

Chapter Five

WHO CHOOSES THE TIME OF DEATH?

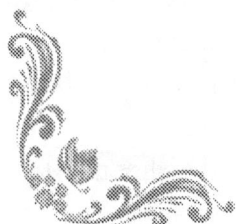

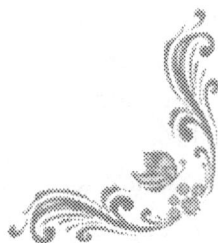

THE LITTLE MAN

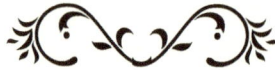

There was something that I found really helped me in dealing with the families, and I just seemed to do it naturally. It was that every patient I had was someone's father or mother, sister or brother, aunt or uncle, or child. I have all of those and can relate on that level.

One day I was going to see this little man whom I had been seeing for a while. His daughter's name was Jan. She was probably about 10 years older than I, but immediately she was very warm to me. Of course, I put myself in her situation. She was taking care of her dad in her home. She moved him up from south Florida. I will just refer to him as the "little man."

He was diagnosed with cancer, but he really didn't have a lot of problems with symptom control. I was one of the few people he'd allow to talk to him. He was just so cute. He decided one day that shark cartilage was going to help him. Well, you know, I hate for people to tell me what to do and what not to do, so I said, "Okay, take shark cartilage." I thought, well, it might work and it might not. Quite honestly, when I had a 4+ Pap Smear[17] (which ended up being a little false alarm) I tried it, too! You just never know.

Jan was working at home and her husband worked nights and slept soundly during the day. She was a very attentive caregiver and her father loved her very much. I visited every week, and the little man was getting weaker. His main problem was lack of appetite. He was down to drinking about two cans of Ensure[18] a day. He started getting so weak that he couldn't get out of bed, but he fought getting a hospital bed. We got him a hospital bed anyway, because he needed it, and Jan especially needed it as a caretaker.

This man taught me one important thing—and that is why he is in this book. I learned that even when someone is in a coma, you still keep the side-rails up. For all intents and purposes, he was a total care patient. Jan would just turn him and bathe him in bed, as he was unresponsive.

On one of my visits Jan said, "Do you know where I found him last night? I put the side-rail down because I knew he wouldn't go anywhere." When she had heard the door open, she had run to see what was happening, and there he was. She had found him butt-naked at the door with his car keys in his hand and with a hat on, ready to go out the door.

So the moral of this little story is—if someone is in a coma, even if they are almost dead, you still keep the side-rails up. Always, always!

Another important hint, you don't put your fingers in their mouth. Even in a coma or without teeth, they can chomp one of your fingers off. This is just a bit of extra advice.

One of the people I was orienting was our Reimbursement Specialist, who was also a nurse, but she had not been doing active, hands-on nursing.

She and I went to this man's house toward the end of his life. We went over in the morning and he was in the bedroom, comatose. His eyes were semi-open and his breathing had "that sound." It sounds as if the person were breathing in an aquarium, but not so noisily. It is a very faint, wet sound. Not a big gurgling or anything, but very faint. Once you have heard it a few times, it is very distinctive.

He had that sound, so I knew it was close, and I thought he might pass while we were standing there. The other nurse and I prepared Jan for what was to come.

The nurse and I went to see other patients, but we came back about noon. Something told me that Jan needed a little support, and I wanted to "tuck her in." He was still "Cheyne-Stoking"[19] and I don't know how the man was still alive. His eyelids were semi-open, but his eyes were rolled up a little bit, like he was looking up. We stayed about an hour and then left again to see other patients.

At the end of the work day, I said to the other nurse, "Let's stop in and see Jan one last time today." We popped into the patient's room.

I was standing there looking at him and all of a sudden this little man's eyes opened WIDE. I said, "Jan, come in the room." When she came in, her dad still had his eyes wide open, and the expression on his face was like he was watching a great movie. He smiled—the look on his face! He was not aware of us. He was looking at something beyond. We watched him and he turned his head toward Jan with this peaceful look on his face, and a smile, and his eyes wide open. I knew the angels were beautiful. You could tell by the look on his face—pure unadulterated joy.

When he took his last breath, his eyes were open looking at Jan. That's when I realized that people choose who they want to be present when they die. That little man didn't want Jan by herself. He loved his daughter. She thought she could handle it, but he wanted to be sure that we were there for her.

I'm being perfectly open with you, because I want you to know these emotions are very natural. I started crying, because I had never seen anything like this before. It was like when I had watched babies being born. I cry every time I see a baby being born. I cry every time a person dies.

His spirit left, and it was so beautiful. The nurse I was orienting was consoling me! That was funny. So we waited a while for the funeral home people to come and everything to settle down. It was one of my first deaths, and it was beautiful.

And remember—NEVER put the side-rails down! Not for ONE minute, no matter what the patient's condition!

MRS. ANDREWS

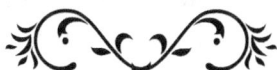

*H*ave you ever walked into a house and met somebody you just loved immediately? Just like you have always known them and there is an instant kinship? Well that's pretty much what happened with this patient of mine—I'll call her Mrs. Andrews.

When I first met Mrs. Andrews it was like I'd known her my whole life. She was probably in her late 60's. She and her husband were living with her daughter in a very, very nice home. She had this huge, huge abdomen. She had just been diagnosed with pancreatic cancer, and she was little orange at the time.

She said, "I can't believe it. They just told me I had cancer and walked out of the room. Some nurse came in and told me to go to Hospice, and here I am."

So I started from ground zero explaining about Hospice, my role in her care, and the additional resources available. I kept thinking, there could be a better way to tell her. And yet, she was just love personified. She had all these children and grandchildren whom she loved dearly, and they loved her.

In the end, she taught me a wonderful lesson, but initially our weekly visits mainly centered on her nausea and vomiting. She would throw up. I would call the doctor, and he would prescribe something for it. We would start the regime. It would work for a couple of days, and then it would stop working. I would go back to the doctor and we'd try different combinations of anti-emetics. We finally found out that she had developed a blockage. Keeping her bowels open was pretty difficult, so the vomiting was a result of the blockage.

I remember one day I went to their house toward the end of the day and I had a migraine headache. She was in a guest room where she and her husband stayed. They had these darling little twin beds and it was decorated like a kid's room. She was lying in bed with a cloth on her forehead and had a bucket next to her. She had been throwing up and felt terrible.

I walked in and tried to sit on the side of the bed, and she said, "Honey, you don't look good."

I said, "I don't feel good at all."

She said, "Well, why don't you lay down on the other bed?"

So I lay down on the other twin bed and asked my "nurse questions," and my migraine just got worse. Her daughter, bless her heart, walked in and saw we were both in very bad shape. She brought me my own bucket and rag. I was barfing into my bucket. Mrs. Andrews was barfing into her bucket. We must have been a sight!

I realize that when I have a symptom or I'm feeling sick, it makes me even more compassionate towards the patient. I think sometimes that's why I'm plagued with headaches after my car accident, headaches and nausea. I think it gives me more compassion for people with these symptoms. When someone has nausea, I will be on a doctor like a hound dog to do something to help that person. We are talking about going to any length, because I understand the discomfort from personal experience.

I'm not saying that the things that I don't have, I don't tend to—because I do. But I think it is a very human thing that I was lying there throwing up and in pain and she was lying there throwing up from pain, so I wanted to relieve that pain quickly.

I had no medication with me, but as soon as my stomach was empty and the visit was over, I called the doctor and got her on some Ativan[20]—a large dose of it—for the nausea. We had already tried

Compazine, Phenergan, and even Dramamine[21]. We had tried suppositories. We had tried Zofran[22]. We would use combinations of them—nothing worked. So Ativan was prescribed. The courier was walking up to the house with the prescription when I was leaving. I just prayed that it would work.

When I walked up to my car door, I realized my keys were locked in my car. It was like the perfect ending to the day. I went back into the house, called my "significant other," and lay down. This family is a family who really includes everybody, and it was so nice to see that God takes care of each of us. The long story, short—I got to give her the first dose of Ativan, and her nausea and vomiting stopped. It was wonderful.

Time went on with this little lady, and her obstruction got to the point where she had to be hospitalized as she started to die. I didn't think it was a good plan to have her in the home when she died, because her daughter had to work. She didn't really have a full-time caregiver. Her husband was very elderly and was not able to handle everything. She had six children and many relatives, but none were able to be full-time caregivers. So she was put in the hospital.

She was talking less, getting lethargic, and losing some level of consciousness. She was getting a little more confused, and then she started talking to people who we couldn't see—like "Momma." And you know that when people start talking to their deceased momma, that's when the time is close.

So I started teaching the family about signs and symptoms of the dying process. Each family member (I think there were a million!) read "The Better Fight"—that was the pamphlet available at the time. Mrs. Andrews was only getting IV morphine and IV Ativan at the time. She had stopped eating. Her body had pretty much shut down. She became incontinent, and then she just withdrew completely. That was about the fourth day she was in the hospital.

The fifth day, I was preparing the family, because her blood pressure was low and her heart rate high. She was not communicating with anyone. Her eyes were rolled back in her head. She looked, to all intents and purposes, like she was dying. People ask me all the time, "When?" Well, as you know and I know—only God knows. But people need some idea. So my "good rule of thumb" is, without anything to eat or drink—and that means no sips, no licks, no lollypops, no drips, no nothing, no food or liquid, nothing for 2 to 72 hours—that's the time frame in most cases. And then along came Mrs. Andrews to blow my theory.

By this time there were 10 people—6 children and 4 grandchildren—camping out in the room. It was a private room, fortunately. Sleeping bags were all over the floor. Sometimes I didn't even know there were other people in the room, because they were on the floor on the other side of the bed. Then all of a sudden I would see a person's head stick up. She always had family in the room, and I thought she would go very soon.

The sixth day came. I walked in and started to talk to them. I wondered if everybody had said everything they needed to say to her. So I had The Talk with all of them, every single one of them. The talk was that they needed to let Mama know that they were going to be okay. The husband, especially, needed to tell Mrs. Andrews that he was going to be okay. They needed to map it out for her. That was their assignment.

People get very, very tired of hanging around and waiting, and they feel guilty for those thoughts. After being in a hospital seven days and seven nights, and sleeping over, and always being there—waiting, and waiting, doing everything possible—their emotions were just under a rug. They had gone from highs to lows. These people had really been through it.

The eighth day came. I walked in. She was still there. They had all told her it was okay to go, and they looked at me as if to ask, why is she still alive? I did not have a clue.

I went in on the ninth day. These people had become like family to me by this time. They barely gave me a glance—like, yeah, yeah, it's just you. I thought there had to be a reason she was hanging on. Then we remembered that she had a disabled child. This child was now an adult and functional, but she really didn't understand the whole concept of what was happening. I felt sure that Mrs. Andrews was waiting for her "baby" to tell her that she would be okay.

So I took the "baby" down to the cafeteria, and we had a heart-to-heart. We were sure that was IT. THAT was the missing link right there! So this gal, who had some learning disabilities and some mental problems, went up to Mrs. Andrews' room. She wanted her older sister in the room with her. There was always SOMEONE in the room. She told Mama exactly how she was going to be okay. The older sister and the "baby" of the family mapped it out for her. We were all sure THAT was the ticket. Then everybody came back into the room, and waited for Mrs. Andrews to die peacefully, now that we had covered every base.

Day 10 came and Mrs. Andrews was STILL alive. I walked in—nobody, I mean nobody, even got up. Everybody just stayed on the floor, and they looked at me like, what now? I was at a total loss.

There were always so many people in this room. They would sit on the bed and would reminisce. They would party, and they would call in for food and eat. Basically, they were LIVING in this room, just like in a hotel room, and after a while, they kind of forgot about Mrs. Andrews.

Then came day 11, day 12, day 13, and day 14. Now by this time, I was going every two days, because they were sure I didn't know what I was talking about. I was even wondering if I knew what I talking about!

On the fifteenth day, I decided to save Mrs. Andrews for my last visit. So I walked in around five o'clock that afternoon.

I said, "Hey, Mrs. Andrews. It's good to see you."

I talked to everybody there. There were about three kids there. I left with no change in the patient.

About nine o'clock that night, I got the phone call. Mrs. Andrews had died. Do you know when she died? Of the three people in the room when I left, two of them went down to the cafeteria and one of them went to make a phone call down the hall. So, for the first time in 15 days—the FIRST TIME—Mrs. Andrews was totally alone. And she died.

I learned that people choose how they want to die, with whom they want to die, and that sometimes they just want to be alone. I've noticed this even more over time, but she was one of my earlier experiences. A lot of mothers, especially, don't want anyone with them when they die. So I always encourage people to give them space. Give people time alone. Say what you need to say, but give them time alone as well.

Mrs. Andrews taught me, and a lot of other people, an invaluable lesson. More important, it really brings it home how when I am with a person as they die—how truly, truly honored I feel. And how truly honored you should feel. But if you are not there when they die, it's simply because that is what that person wants. I think dying is such a personal experience, that people should have it any way they want. Mrs. Andrews wanted to be alone; that was her choice.

SHANA

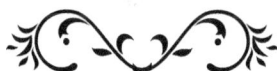

I need to tell you about a woman named Shana. She was 41 years old and a Messianic Jew. She was a beautiful, beautiful, strong woman. I met this lady and spent a couple of hours with her on the first visit. After doing her physical assessment, we prayed together. It just clicked; I felt different and she felt different.

As time went on, I began seeing her once a week. She had lung cancer. When I listened to her lungs with the stethoscope, I heard decreasing air exchange as the weeks went by. I frequently talked to the Hospice physician—called almost every time I was there—and we would change her medication. She was very verbal about her physical condition. Then we would pray. I always felt renewed after seeing her, and I never wanted to leave.

Sometimes our prayer time was specifically for me. When it was for her, it was always about being more comfortable with God while in her apartment, because with very little air exchange, she was unable leave her apartment after about a week. She had been used to doing her ministry in an outbound way. She was very action-oriented. She had many friends, and staying in her home was very difficult for her. But as her physical condition declined, she could maneuver better at home, because she was on oxygen.

As time went on, more of our prayers became centered on being comfortable just BEING. That is something I have struggled with my whole life. I don't know where I got the impression that I'm a human "doing." but Shana reminded me that I am a human BEING. So our prayers were very concentrated on her being more comfortable and feeling worthy of being on this planet and doing service to God. That was her desire—without leaving her house, with just spending time with God.

I will never forget those times that we prayed. It became very clear to me that we are all "okay" and it is all right that we take up space on this planet, even if we never DO a single thing. Even if we just ARE—period—God loves us. We are his children. We were created for companionship for him. So she became more comfortable with "being," but she had to fight that human desire to be out there busy "doing."

As I mentioned, sometimes our prayer times were for me. Her cat wanted to be all over me. When I told her I was highly allergic to cats, she laid her hands on me while we were praying and prayed that I would be healed of my allergies to cats. I never had a single problem after that.

There were so many times that I would go to see her, and I would just want to "do" so much for her. She couldn't clean her apartment after a while and it really bothered her. Our social worker had attempted to get a homemaker to do her housecleaning, but it just kept falling through. This really discouraged her. Vacuuming isn't a thing that a Hospice nurse does. However, I felt the strongest pull to vacuum her house for her.

I was talking to a friend of mine, who was trying to become less self-centered, and he wanted to go help her, too. So we got our cleaning supplies and went over one night. We were there about three hours, and we scrubbed her bathrooms as if they were our own. I vacuumed. He worked in the shower stalls. We cleaned that house so that she would be comfortable. And you know, it was an honor.

My friend and I got a lot out of serving her in this way. She always found it difficult to ask people to help her. She looked at my friend and said, "You know, you have a lovely way of helping without making me feel uncomfortable about it." I guess it was kind of a backward compliment, but it was truly sweet and special. I would do it again in a heartbeat. It helped both of us to grow.

As time went on, Shana was able to do less and less. She could go from her window to her chair in the living room, and from her chair in her living room to her bed. That was her limit.

I often felt I was walking on holy ground when I entered Shana's house. During our second-to-the-last prayer session, after I had completed her physical assessment, I had this vision that Shana was on the altar of God right there in her little apartment. That WAS the altar of God. Every time she asked Him for something or even approached Him, He was right there attending to her every thought. She didn't have to struggle into grace like I do. I can be on my knees for half an hour before I feel like I'm in the presence of God or that He is even paying attention. I know that's not true, but that's how I feel. But this woman would just think about God, and He would be right there. And I saw it!

She became more and more comfortable with herself, simply being on this earth to be a companion to God. Just to be. And that was a major transformation. That taught me SO much about self-worth. A lot of us base our self-worth on what we do, and that really shouldn't be. We are supposed to base our self-worth, according to the Bible, on how much faith God has given us. And we can ask for more faith! So our self-worth is basically up to us and not based on our accomplishments or what we do.

My routine for going to see Shana was to go in, sit down with her, do a physical assessment, talk to the doctor, and then regroup and pray with her. Then I would leave. Usually, our visits took a couple hours, and I always felt like I had been in the presence of God.

I was orienting a new Hospice nurse, a strong Christian woman, and we went to see Shana. Shana was short of breath, just sitting there, with no exertion. She got up to go to the window with the help of the new nurse, but barely made it back to her chair. It looked like she was really declining. I could hear NO air exchange in her lungs, so I called our physician. I explained to him what was going on, giving the physical assessment—I could not hear fluid in her lungs, so we couldn't diurese[23] her. She was already on steroids and was sleeping a lot. Her appetite, of course, was not good, and it had decreased even more.

I will never forget sitting up at the kitchen counter, calling the doctor. The other nurse was sitting with Shana, in another part of the room. I had explained Shana's symptoms and the doctor said, "Patty, I really think that there is nothing more that we can do. I think that, basically, she has run out of air. She is like a car that's run out of gas, and we can't refill it. We can't do anything about it."

Our Hospice physicians are very compassionate. This one, who is a dear friend of mine, picked up on the fact that I was pretty upset about this. I know I was starting to lose my objectivity, because I didn't WANT this woman to die. She had no family nearby that she could call on. She was living alone, and it was extremely sad. I sat there after hanging up with him, and I cried over in the corner very quietly.

After I got myself together, I went to sit with Shana and the other nurse. Shana looked at me, and she knew that I knew something. I just didn't have it in me to sugarcoat anything. I said to her, "Shana, in my opinion and in my best professional judgment, it is not safe for you to be alone anymore. You are basically running out of gas."

Shana looked at me, and she started to cry. Not those horrible tears of revelation that may come the first time someone thinks about dying. No, it was softer, more like concern, like she hurt for me having to tell her. She said softly, "I know. God has prepared me."

Even as I was telling her this, the phone rang. Keep in mind that she had no family in town and had not asked anybody for help. I didn't know who was on the other end of the phone, but her name was Donna. Shana said, "Donna, I need you to come over tonight." Apparently, Donna said that was why she was calling. She was trying to call in while I was on the phone with the doctor, because God told her that she needed to come over and be with Shana.

That to me is so incredible, that God would plant an idea in a person's head to go be with someone at the very moment that they needed it, but God loved Shana so much. I guess, in retrospect, it makes sense!

I talked to Donna on the phone. I told her what the medication regime was, and I wrote it down. We prayed with Shana, and when the other nurse and I left Shana's home, I didn't realize it would be the last time that I saw her. Maybe God was protecting me, or her.

After we left, the other nurse and I talked. She turned to me and said, "I didn't know WHY I came to orient with Hospice, because I thought up to this point that this is really the most terrible occupation anybody could ever choose as a nurse."

After I got off the floor laughing and agreeing with her, she said, "I understand now that this is a mission. This is something that God chooses you to do, and this is what I want to do. Thank you."

I said, "Well, thank Shana." Shana had prayed for us before we left. Amazing!

That was a Friday. I didn't work on Saturday, but I worked the Triage on Sunday—meaning that I was at the other end of the phone when people would call Hospice for all the patients. If they needed a visit I would send out another nurse. So I was working Triage, and I got a call from Shana's sister in New Jersey, asking what was going on. I basically told her, and said she needed to come.

She said, "Well, I can't now. I talked to Shana two days ago, and she understands."

Apparently, Shana had told her on the phone about a week prior that she really didn't need to come, that Shana was okay with everything. She knew where she was going. She was more comfortable with God "out of her body" at that moment than she was "in her body." Her sister was emotional, but was okay with it.

Later I got a call from Donna. Donna asked me questions about the medication, and we talked about Shana. Then I asked to speak to her.

Shana sounded WONDERFUL! She sounded calm and peaceful— a little sleepy, but fine. That was probably at two o'clock in the afternoon.

I called her again about four o'clock, because I was leaving Hospice at six. Shana answered the phone and we talked briefly. She was just wonderful to me. I made sure that she understood about her medications. She still sounded like she was in a dream state—very relaxed, very happy, very calm. Just before hanging up, I asked, "Is Donna handling everything okay?

She said, "Donna is fine. She is going to be staying with me."

I said, "That is just wonderful."

The sound of her voice was so peaceful. She had never said this over the phone to me before, but she said, "I want you to know that I thank you for everything that you are doing, and I really love you."

"I know, Shana," I said, "I love you, too."

There wasn't a sound of finality about anything that she said, but that was the last time I talked to her. Apparently, at about 9:30 or 10:00 that night, Shana was in bed and her friend Donna was next to her. Shana was in a sleeping state, and she simply took her last breath with a slight smile on her face. No struggle or anything. And I thought of the honor I felt at having known and spent time with Shana.

It is so strange to go into someone's house and realize that you are leaving with more spiritual goodies than you brought in to give to your patient. So I consider Shana a sheer gift from God to me. I just know that I grew because God loved me through this person. It was amazing.

It reminded me that, even in the final hours of death that we all will go through, we don't need to fear being alone. God doesn't let that happen. When you love Him, He just makes it all work out. That is a very good lesson.

THE RECLINER LADY

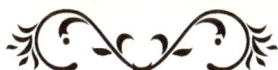

I met a Hospice patient when I was working out at the beach. She was diagnosed with liver cancer and had ascites[24]. Her liver was so swollen, she looked pregnant. This lady could get around a little bit, mostly just from her recliner to her wheelchair. Her husband was not really a caregiver.

This lady wanted to go see her best friend in New York. I honestly don't know how she did it, but she made the arrangements to get to the plane, to be transported in the Atlanta airport to the next plane, and to get to her friend. She stayed for seven days. She came back and sat in her recliner, which she did almost all the time. She loved that recliner.

When I visited her after her return from New York, she was sitting in her recliner with this far away expression on her face. It was almost like she was in "La La Land." Like she was one of those flower children from the '60's, where everything is lovely and beautiful, and they have this "La La" tone to their voice. (You know, when you are in a bad mood you just want to slap them out of it.) But hers was very real. It was just like she was in this state of "Everything was beautiful there; I had a good time with my friend; I am totally at peace."

Her vital signs were stable. Her husband was not really in the picture. He was there physically, but he wasn't really there as a comforter and supporter. I told him that if she wanted to stay in the recliner she could. She would get up a couple of times a day and change her Depends[25] herself, very slowly—even though I had taught her husband how to do this.

She died the very next day. People do what they need to do before they die. She needed to see her friend in New York. So I learned from that—not only that people do what they need to do, but also to trust your instincts. My first thought when I saw her, was that she was dying. Yet her vital signs were fine. So I assumed my instinct was wrong.

I have learned to always trust my gut feelings. If you come to Hospice, and you feel like it's just the most natural, normal thing for you to take care of dying people, to teach them the dying process, and you really don't have a problem with it—then you are chosen.

And if you are chosen, God will tell you when someone is dying. He will give you that instinct. I have flat-out asked Him, "Is this person dying?" And when He said, "Yes," I intentionally do not believe Him. And then they die, and I remember He tried to tell me. So, trust your gut. Because if you have been called to this, as I was, He won't steer you wrong. He wants you to prepare these people. He wants YOU to be ready, and He wants you to do what is best for patients and their families.

So this lady died in her recliner, and she was quite happy. But the people from the funeral home had quite a time. This is what you run into when people die in precarious positions. And, speaking of that situation, I had another patient... Well, I guess I'll just go on into it... I had this little patient that lived by himself and insisted on it. This is a whole different story by the way. I'll name him Jim...

JIM

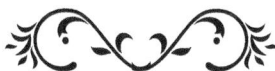

I can't remember his actual name, but he was just darling. The social worker and I worked with him together, because he was so young. He would go into the bathroom in the middle of the night and sometimes would fall asleep on the toilet.

One morning I got a call from Terry, his home health aide, saying that he told her that he had fallen off the toilet the night before, because he got so sleepy.

Well, I didn't take it too seriously. I guess I sometimes get in the state of mind that some people are going to live forever in this program. Talk about MY denial, right?

So, to make a long story short, Jim was in the bathroom in the middle of the night and apparently died on the toilet, which was where they found him the next day. According to the Report, he had apparently been there for hours so he had kind of stiffened up in that position—kind of like Rodin's sculpture, "The Thinker." Rigor mortis had set in.

This isn't funny, but this is Hospice humor. When they put him on the stretcher, I can just imagine that he was kind of curled up like a little creature. You know, with his elbow on his knee and his hand under his chin. I know this isn't funny, but we at Hospice do just have a bizarre sense of humor, and you really have to, in order to deal with the heavier issues.

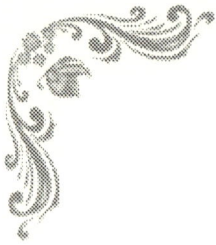

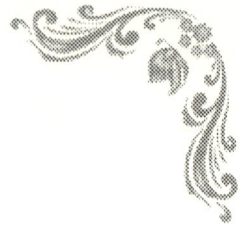

Chapter Six

THE BITTERSWEET

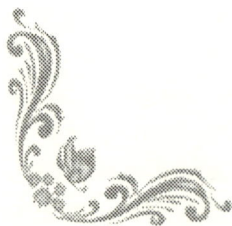

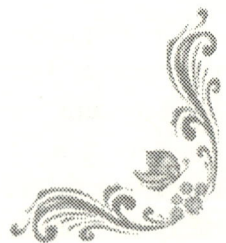

GINNY

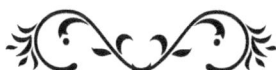

Ginny lived down the street from me in an assisted living facility. I always told her, "Hey, if I was 55 years old, I'd move out of my condo and move in right next door to you." It was great there! She lived by herself, but very comfortably.

When I first met her, she opened the door looking healthier than I did. She was walking around very capably. She was well-dressed. She had these sparkly blue eyes, and was so full of the joy.

I said, "Are you sure that you should be in Hospice?"

She said, "Well, yeah."

I did request her X-rays to verify she had lung cancer. When I looked at her X-rays, I saw the tumors in her lungs were very large. I honestly could not hear breathing sounds with my stethoscope from the very start. I listened intently for them. I would have her stand up, sit down, lie down, you name it, and I could hear nothing. There was zero airflow, but this lady was more alive than I ever hope to be. The only other medical problem that she ever had was with her bowels—which we controlled with Senokot and Haley's MO[26]—great stuff!

Our conversations basically evolved during lunch. She took me to lunch every week. We would do her physical assessment and review her medications prior to eating. She would say, "Now when the time comes to go to the Hospice Center…" (This is an inpatient center—

24 beds. It's beautiful—the Ritz Carlton of hospices.) "…When the time comes, I want you to tell me and don't be afraid. Just tell me."

So I agreed that I would.

She was at high risk for bleed out[27], so we had a plan. If she started coughing up blood, she would call me, she would unlock the door, she would take her Valium, and she would sit down and stay calm. She understood it, and she had no fear of death—none. She had a darling little granddaughter who would sometimes come and eat lunch with us too. Ginny became my friend and my prayer partner.

After a period of time—I worked with her for about nine months—she did start to get weaker. I said, "You know, Ginny, while you've got the time and while you are still moving around, we should go visit the Hospice Center."

She did, and she loved it. "Better sooner than later," she said. I agreed with her.

She had another X-ray taken of her lungs. The tumors had grown. I still heard nothing—no airflow through her lungs. So she went to live at the Hospice Center.

Well, Ginny got better. She became a Hospice volunteer. I would walk into one of the conference rooms and see all of these volunteers stuffing envelopes, and there would be Ginny. She did a lot of good things for the people at the Hospice Center. Nobody could believe that she was a patient!

I just can't help but smile while I'm telling you about her. She was one of those people who would always ask you, "Well, how are you doing?" and really want to know the answer. She was very involved in my life. I told her everything. She started going to my church. Everybody loved her. She had been a member of Hope Baptist Church. So she named my church Little Hope Baptist Church. She was just a hoot.

Soon Ginny grew very weak, and she started dying. Everybody in the Hospice Center was so sad, oh, my gosh. We prepared her family. Then, a week later, she came out of it better than ever. She was walking around and seemed to be doing fine!

One day she decided that she really wanted to be on the Monday Night Live Football Show, so she went over to one of the local sports bars—and they put her on TV. There was a sports announcer there and Ginny told him she wanted to talk to one of the local football players.

They put her in the recliner, and the sports announcer came up to her and said, "Well, Ginny. Ginny is our Hospice patient, and Ginny, we heard that you were just dying to get here." This poor man didn't say this on purpose, but when he realized what he had said, he was so embarrassed.

She looked at him and patted his hand, and she said, "That's okay honey. It's going to happen to all of us." She was just such a joy.

On another occasion, Ginny went up in a hot air balloon with another Hospice patient; this was written up in the newspaper. She did so many things. She started hanging around with a little lady who was her neighbor at the Hospice Center, and they became best friends. When this little lady died, it probably occurred to Ginny that she might really be a Hospice patient.

While Ginny was in the Hospice Center, I was a field nurse. They call those of us who go to the homes "out house" nurses, because the "in house" nurses are the ones at the Hospice. She always thought that was so funny.

I would visit her often at the Hospice Center. The second to last time I saw her, she was sitting in her reclining chair, her eyes were as clear as crystal, and she was very weak. She could no longer stand by herself.

She said, "Hello, how are you? I'm doing fine for the condition I'm in. I'm getting ready to go. God is with me."

I had taken a friend of mine with me that day, and he was very close to tears, as he was touched by her wonderful attitude. It is still hard for some people to be around those who are dying. She was physically comfortable—but getting progressively weaker.

I was overwhelmed with paperwork at the time, so I went to the Hospice one day and sat next to her bed, working. Her room was decorated just like her room at the home—very comfortably. She had been in the Hospice Center for a year, and everyone was grieving because Ginny was dying.

She was pretty non-responsive by this time. She hadn't said a word in two days. She hadn't eaten anything in two days. All of a sudden I looked up, and she was looking right at me. At the same time, we said to each other, "Hey, pretty girl." And we just started to laugh. I laughed hysterically. She was just laughing as much as a person in a semi-coma can, and I got to tell her I loved her.

She was truly a role model to me. No matter how you are leaving this world and how much you will miss people, you can still be interested in others, and THAT is the joy of life. I will never forget Ginny. She was one of the people who have taught me about life. I just hope I have half of her grace when I leave, for Ginny was my friend.

RUTH

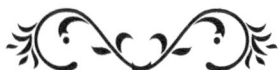

I want to tell you about a person named Ruth. I just loved Ruth and her husband, Frank. She had ovarian cancer. These people were about the age of my parents—early 70's. Going to visit them every week was a joy. It was funny—I couldn't go at two o'clock, since Ruth watched "Law and Order" at that time. So I would visit her another time so we could talk.

This was when I met a TRUE hero. Frank, her husband, had been a prison of war and had written a book about it. He gave me a copy and I read it. That book was the most amazing thing I had read about a human being whom I had actually met. Once again, it's the people that you meet that make this job worthwhile. We just had a great time.

After a while, Ruth had some lab work done, and her blood work showed that her cancer had gone into remission. All her church family prayed for her and she actually got better. I discharged her from the Hospice program, and then my territory changed, so I lost track of her.

About a year later I heard that she was in the Hospice Center, so I went to see her. She had had a "great year off" from Hospice, and I enjoyed hearing her stories. She had created some great memories.

Ruth and Frank were neat people, and I am glad they got an extra year together.

GERALD GRAYSON

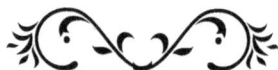

*T*here are many patients and their families who have
helped me to grow spiritually. There is one such person
I want to tell you about—Gerald Grayson. Gerald was
my patient and his wife's name was Christine.

You know it's strange, but when a person has a strong spiritual life,
it makes a difference in the way they die. It's like God is able to prepare these people better. I guess the moral of this lovely man's story is
to "prepare." Get to know your Maker early. It's like investing time in
a long-term relationship.

The first time I went to see Gerald and Christine, I noticed there
was a sense of peace. They lived in a beautiful condominium overlooking the river. When I met Christine, she was sparkly-eyed and full
of faith. She was a beautiful woman.

Then I talked to Gerald, and he was just a sweet man. He had cancer and also a bit of Alzheimer's. He always answered "Yes," and he'd
laugh a little. Each visit with him was a delight. He really had no pain.
We battled his urinary infections, because he had a Foley catheter.
Mainly, we dealt with little things that would come up, like respirato-
ry infections. He built up a lot of fluid in his body, so diuresing him
was a daily monitoring process.

94

As Gerald declined, it was difficult because he moved from a chair to a wheelchair, and then from a wheelchair to getting in and out of bed. We got a bed for him and put it up in the den with the big screen TV, so people could come visit him. He was always so pleasant and sweet, but very emotional. Whenever he would talk about God, "our incredibly loving all-powerful Creator" (these are his words) he would cry. They weren't tears of sadness, but tears of awe. You could just see that his relationship with God was so real.

I will never forget one visit when I was listening to his lungs. Christine was there and also a few family friends. The bed was pretty well cranked up, and Gerald grabbed my hand. He wasn't talking very much, but he looked over at me and said, "I love you" with so much meaning. He took my hand. He kissed it, and said, "Jesus loves you." It was so weird—he and I just started singing "Jesus Loves Me." We weren't singing to each other—I don't know who we were singing to—but there was just a wonderful, wonderful feel to that room. There was peace.

The Grayson's had a nephew from out-of-town. I believe he was a fireman. He was a big hefty guy, so he could turn Gerald (who was no small person) and take care of him. The love shown toward this man was so overwhelming. It was such a privilege and an honor to be able to serve this family. I kept thinking, God, who am I to even be in the presence of these spiritual giants?

During Gerald's illness, a hurricane was predicted to hit the coast in our area. The Graysons were up on the "millionth" floor in their condo overlooking the water, so we made preparations. We got oxygen and a generator, because they knew that they couldn't move him due to his size and their location in the high-rise.

I also needed to prepare my own house, but I stopped over at a local barbeque restaurant on the way home to have lunch. It is the strangest thing how God brings people together. There was this nice looking couple in the back of the restaurant. I looked at the man, and he looked JUST like Gerald—it was unreal.

"You look just like Gerald Grayson!" I said.

"That's because I'm Gerald Grayson, Jr.!" he replied.

They invited me to join them for lunch. We talked about preparing for the hurricane. Everybody had bought plywood for sealing windows, and drinking water. I was planning to head over to the Hospice Center to answer the phones as soon as I made sure my daughter was safe. We talked about Gerald and Christine, and I came to know his son and his wife. I talked to them about the dying process and about how his dad was all right with it—his dad was just fine. It was very special.

Gerald died very peacefully. Christine wrote the most beautiful letter to her friends at Christmas—a little testimony. There was a big funeral for him at the Baptist church. While I was on my way to the church, I was paged. I had to go see another patient, so I thought—well, I'll get to the graveside service.

After I had seen my patient and was arriving at the graveside, I got paged again. Sometimes public closure is just not meant to be, but I did have personal closure with him. I know where he is—and what a beautiful person he is—what an absolutely beautiful person. I guess, in some ways, I'm having my closure now.

It is hard to think back about these people who have touched my life. So many heroes are dying off. I know God will send some new heroes—people to show other people the way. When you are called to do Hospice work, you get into very intense, close relationships with people. The real difficulty comes after they are gone. You've built these relationships, but you have to keep moving on. You have to go on and serve other people.

There seems to be not enough time to keep up with all these folks. Since Gerald died, Christine and I keep saying we will get together. We have actually run into each other several times. I do feel bad about that—not having enough time to see her and the other people who mean so much to me.

I hope these folks will truly understand that I love them and always will. I did give them my very best. My thoughts and my prayers are always with them. It was such an honor to know each and every one.

I say to my parents whenever I leave them, "You know, if I leave you and get hit by a bus, don't be sad. I will see you in heaven." And that's how I feel about pretty much everybody.

It is really nice to be able to spend time with people that you love. But it's such an odd feeling to have these relationships formed on such a deep level, and then not have contact with these people again. I will always remember singing, "Jesus Loves Me" with Gerald.

JEFFREY

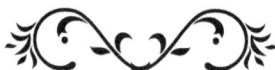

As I sat on the beach early one morning, watching the sun come up, I saw an older man, very frail, out there with a pitch fork picking up the seaweed and putting it in a bucket. Somehow, it reminded me of Jeffrey.

Jeffrey and I met when his wife came into the Hospice program. I went over to his big house on the river, and he was there with his wife, who had a diagnosis of nutritional marasmus[28]. She also had dementia and was in need of total care. Jeffrey, about 80 years old, was very slender and hunched over, though if he had stood up straight, he would have been nearly six feet tall. He was assisting—nearly carrying—his wife from the bed to the bedside commode. When he got her back to bed and walked away, all you heard was her calling "Jeffrey… Jeffrey…" That's what she did all day long, just call for him to come and take care of her in some way.

And that is just what Jeffrey did all day—take care of Rebecca. He watched Rebecca. He would put her into the wheelchair and wheel her into the kitchen. They would sit there, and he would encourage her to sip some orange juice. He had been doing this for the previous three years before I met him.

Rebecca's doctor recommended that she become a Hospice patient. The doctor loved this couple so much, he begged Rebecca to eat something because she was starving herself to death. But sometimes, with dementia, you can't expect people to respond.

So I would visit Jeffrey and Rebecca, but basically I felt helpless. I would say, "Jeffrey, what can I do for you?"

"Well, there is really nothing you can do," he would say. "I take care of her, I don't really need anything."

Rebecca started to stay up all night. When I saw Jeffrey, he always looked so tired. He was up all night with her—up and down, on and off that bedside commode, changing her, taking care of her. He traded out their king-size bed for one of those beds that separate in the middle and move into various positions. That way he could make the beds easier and he felt she would be more comfortable.

Our visits really consisted of me listening to him tell me how he was up all night taking care of her. It would just break my heart. I asked, "Jeffrey, can't we get somebody to come help you?"

But he would just say no. Jeffrey wanted to take care of Rebecca himself. Over time I began to learn the depth of this man. I learned about the things he had done in his life, the incredible person he was and continued to be through his wife's illness and death—week after week.

He finally allowed me to get somebody to come stay with him at night—just a couple nights a week. Jeffrey insisted that these folks claim Social Security. He said if they didn't, and he didn't take out taxes, how would they support themselves later on? He was always concerned about other people.

Once I went to the house, and Jeffrey was turning Rebecca, who was skin and bones by this time. We were sitting alongside the bed, and he was telling me how he rubbed her feet, and how he got her into the shower on a shower chair and bathed her. He turned to me with these huge eyes (his eyes were like a 45-year-old man in an 80-year-old body), and he said, "Yeah, I gave her a bath." And he kind of chuckled and said, "I sure wish she would have let me do this when she was younger. It could have been fun." Apparently, Rebecca was a very private person. She would even go into the closet to get dressed. This was the first glimpse Jeffrey gave me of his fun side.

Jeffrey gave me a check for $2,000 made out to Hospice on one occasion. I took the check to Hospice and logged the donation. The next week I was in my car leaving his house and noticed a check peeking out of my paperwork. It was a check for $1,000 made out to ME. I was only two blocks from his house so I turned around and took the check back to him. I thought it was going to break his heart when I said, "Jeffrey, I can't accept this. As a Hospice employee, that would not be ethical."

He said, "But I want YOU to have it. Hospice got their money. This is for you."

I said, "I'm so sorry. I just can't accept this."

He said, "You've been my right-hand man. We have worked together."

I never realized how he felt before that, because he had asked for so little. Bottom line, I didn't take the money. Ethics rule #1: If a family offers something to eat or drink and it is in your stomach when you leave, it is fine. Otherwise, don't accept anything and don't take money unless it is a Hospice donation.

Jeffrey loved taking care of Rebecca. That was his life. They had lived a very good life. She had been his bookkeeper for his business. They had a nice home, and he had bought her the very first Corvette, which was her pride and joy.

One morning I woke up, and I just had them both on my mind. I guess it was about 8:40 A.M. when my pager went off with Jeffrey's number. I called him, and he said, "Please come now." He was totally beside himself—Rebecca had died.

So I went to the house, and his housekeeper let me in. I walked back to the bedroom that I had walked back to so many times before, and Jeffrey was sitting on the side of the bed holding Rebecca's hand. He was just doubled over with grief, crying. I went over and just sat with him. I put my arm around him, and we both cried. Then he said something that I never before realized, about how a caregiver could feel. He looked over at me and said, "I can't believe that I let her down...that I left her."

I thought—this man has lost him mind! But then I could see how some caregivers could start getting this weird idea. And I said, "Jeffrey, you have done everything for Rebecca. You have been there day and night and have taken care of her like no one I've ever seen. You didn't leave her. If anything, she left you. Not in a bad sense, but it was time for her to go. But you did not leave her."

And he nodded his head. He cried...I cried...I stayed with him. The neighbors came. The arrangements had already been made. The funeral home came. I drove away a different person.

I have maintained a friendship with Jeffrey. He is an incredible person. He has taught me a lot about the stock market—what to invest in, what not to invest in. This man has built some of our major airports. He has designed and built whole neighborhoods, apartment complexes. He is a very smart man and he taught me a lot about money, and about people, and about love.

Author's Note: Jeffrey has begun a new life with a very special woman. Hope springs eternal.

ETHAN

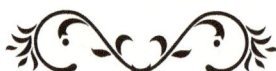

*have put off telling this story because Ethan was so near and dear to my heart and also to the social worker working with me on this case.

Ethan did not want to be in Hospice. When I arrived at the house, I saw this man sitting at the window of his home, using his oxygen and smoking a cigarette. He had so many physical problems. He had major heart problems—an enlarged heart. I don't know how it was still able to maintain his body. Our first visit was basically "shooting the breeze," because he didn't want to talk about Hospice. He and his wife were big golfers, so we could talk about that. This man just became so dear to me. Week after week, I would go to their home and he was the high point of my day. We would talk, and he would tell me his philosophy of life.

As time went on, he had massive breathing troubles. He had chronic obstructive pulmonary disorder (COPD). He also had cancer, but it was really the enlarged heart that was his main problem. He did not want to be a burden on his wife (who is a great friend of mine to this day). They were relatively young—early 60's. He would send her out to work, because he didn't want her around all day worrying about him.

He and I would sit at the table and talk, and we played "word of the day." This is where I got my love for new words. He would ask me if I knew what some unusual word meant. I would say no, and he would tell me—something really wild—and I would take that with me. We talked about everything. He was from England, so I got some history on that as well.

His symptoms were very difficult to control. While our Hospice physician was doing pain and symptomatic management for the cancer, I had to talk to his primary physician for anything that had to do with his heart or the COPD. The doctor was very hard to reach by phone, so one day I actually went to his office and talked to him. He was just stunned and amazed that a Hospice nurse would care so much about a patient. I said, "Well, you know Ethan. How can you not care about him? He has that dry sense of humor." Actually, now that I think about it, Ethan probably put some people off with that dry sense of humor, but I loved it.

Ethan had a hard time getting around because he got so short of breath. His major fear was that he would suffocate. We got some medication that Hospice generally uses for problems like his—but I had to convince his physician it would be a good idea. His physician talked to our physician and found out that we sometimes use concentrated morphine for the symptom of shortness of breath (dyspnea). I convinced him it was a good idea to use it—just a teeny, tiny bit—and it did help.

I had met his wife, Lynn, and his daughter, who was about my age. We would sit and talk openly, and I basically told them what they could expect, to the best of my knowledge. You never know exactly what to expect when it is not a true cancer diagnosis.

My social worker at the time was Allie, and we would both go see him regularly. He became like a surrogate father to us. It was hard to go into his house, as we were both allergic to smoke and he was a heavy smoker. But he was considerate and didn't smoke too much while we were there.

When he started to decline, he would want to go outside and smoke, so we got a wheelchair for him. He just hated equipment that made him less independent, but he had started declining and needed it. He was to the point that he couldn't even stand up and get to his favorite perch in the kitchen, because he had no air capacity.

Lynn finally quit work to stay home with him, and I told her that he was going to go fast. I will never forget the day that he looked at me and said, "Patty, this is no way to live."

He looked terrible, and I told him so.

He said, "I know. Listen, I can't do anything. I'm messing all over myself. I can hardly bring this cigarette to my mouth. This is no way to live. How much longer?"

I took his vital signs. As a medical person, when you're trying to evade your heart, you go to the left-brain activities and do vital signs—at least I have found that to be true for me. His blood pressure was lower. His heart rate was higher. I said, "Ethan, I don't think it's going to be a great deal longer."

He asked, "Will I know what's going on?"

"Well, you're already getting as confused as a bedbug," I said. "Do you know when you're confused?"

He said, "No."

I said, "Well, are you upset about being confused?"

"NO!" he exclaimed. "Because I don't know when I'm confused!"

"Well, this is probably how it will end up for you. You'll just feel like you're floating off. You'll probably start sleeping a lot."

He said, "I'm already sleeping 20 out of 24 hours."

"Case in point," I said.

We were gradually getting more and more care into the home. I had his medications scheduled for daily increases and decreases, and his ability to swallow started to decline. My social worker and I were falling apart at the seams every time we left the house. We started making joint visits, but the last visit we made together, something told me she would not see him again.

She was out of town when he died, and it was difficult for her because she didn't really feel like she had said goodbye. I said, "Oh yeah, you did. He knows. He only had your best interests at heart."

For the last two days he was dying, he was bed-bound. He was, indeed, confused. He did not communicate. We put a draw sheet[29] on his bed to help with turning him, and we got continuous care in the home. We got a wonderful nurse in to take care of him 24/7, because Lynn kept telling me, "Patty! I am not a nurse! I never wanted to be a nurse! You have to do the 'nursey' stuff!"

I said, "Okay, Lynn. I understand."

The last day of his life I visited him in the morning, and he was talking to people we couldn't see. We couldn't really understand what he was saying. He was basically in a comatose state. I put a diaper on him to make sure that Lynn didn't end up with anything she didn't expect, and I just asked her to hold him—just hold him, and she said, "I can do that."

She was afraid, though. She was afraid at first that it would disturb him if she lay next to him. I said, "Lynn you want to let him know that you're here. There is nothing illegal, immoral, or anything else bad about touching a person as they die. It is the most wonderful gift you can give him."

He did die in her arms, for which she was grateful. And that is nursing. That is good nursing. All the technical stuff, basically a trained baboon could do it: the turning, the IVs, and everything else. But for the caring—for that you need a human. You need someone who loves the patient.

After he died, I walked out of the room and burst into tears. This was my first experience of having the family comfort me. He was my buddy, and I knew I would miss him.

Ethan had been a drinker. He would start drinking in the afternoon at four o'clock. So, it got to be five o'clock, and I was "off the pager" and, technically, not working. So while waiting for the funeral home people, we had a toast to Ethan. This was also my first experience drinking with the family. I don't drink very much, but by this time I was pretty distraught. So I thought, why not, and I had a drink with the family.

The funeral home came and went. By this time, we were all indulging in Hospice humor. Lynn was laughing. Her daughter and son-in-law were laughing. We were just toasting Ethan the way that he would have wanted it, because he was a gregarious, funny guy.

When I finally left the house, I wasn't even aware of it, but the one drink had hit home. I drove about a block from the house, pulled off to the side of the road, and took a nap. I woke up an hour later—a little disoriented—and life went on.

Ethan's funeral was held on the river. All of his friends were there, and we shared "Ethan stories." They asked me to talk, and I remembered the one time that I was teaching him how to do an inhaler. So I shared this "nurse" story with a group of non-medical people. This was the funniest experience I have ever had with a patient while teaching them how to use a medical apparatus. I was teaching Ethan how to squirt the little bottle, and when all was said and done and my wonderful instructions had been given, he looked at me and said, in his very English accent, "Now Patty, do I put this in my mouth or up my a__?" It was just an "Ethan" question—hysterical.

As I shared this at his eulogy, I knew without a doubt it was just what he would have wanted—all of his friends around telling funny "Ethan stories." It was great to be able to participate in that. Of course, Allie and I were sitting there holding on to each other, laughing and crying, laughing and crying—and that is just how it goes.

This has been a hard story to tell because, even as I relay this over the tape, I'm crying! I miss him! I really miss him, and a lot of other people do, too!

Lynn and I spend time together, and we talk about him. We talk about the good times, and that's wonderful. I feel like a good friend of mine is gone, but I have gained a friend with Lynn. I don't lose the memories, and it's not hard to see Lynn at all. She is a wonderful friend, and I think that is what I'm most grateful for. Having the opportunity to be a Hospice nurse means that I have met some extraordinary people and have some incredible relationships, for which I am honored. An emotional mess at times—but deeply, deeply honored.

MR. GREEN JEANS

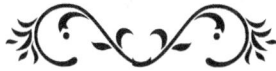

This story is a little unusual because I'm writing about a person who is still living. This story has really been on my mind lately, because I'm on my last two weeks of Hospice work before going PRN[30] and starting school.

This is about a little old man I went to see tonight. However, I did not visit this patient at his home—I went to a bar with a dance floor and karaoke to see him. This is a man I had seen many times over the past years before he became my patient.

Last night when I took Report, I got a message from the assessment nurse. She said, "I am admitting a patient of yours. He's an entertainer every Friday night at a local restaurant club, a standup comedian. He is such a cute, little old man. He's about 80 years old."

This man flashed before my eyes. Over the years, I have gone to that club and seen this odd, little old man. He had a top hat, black suit, gaudy tie, black and white shoes, and sunglasses. He was always dancing with the young girls and partying, and I thought, "That's him. That's my new patient."

The first time I went to his house, I wasn't sure. But as I began talking to him, I thought, "Yes, that is him—top hat and all." We talked, and as I sat in his kitchen, he started revealing to me some profound things.

For example, when he was 50, he was taken out of a deep sleep and found himself standing in the dark. He saw a light. He said it was the most compassionate, comfortable, loving, all-knowing light, and he knew it was God. God asked him a question, which was, "What have you done with what I've given you?" Not in a condemning way, but just asking a question.

When he came back to his body, he thought about the vision and asked God, "What do You want me to do with my life? What is it that You want me to do with what You've given me?"

After giving it some thought, this little man decided, at 50 years of age, to work with disabled people and get them jobs. He only had a high school diploma, and the job descriptions that he wrote were for people with college degrees. He is an amazing person—just an amazing person. He went on to help others and always gave whatever he could.

He also talked to me about our legacies. Legacies, as in—what do we want to leave behind on this earth? That question haunted me. We talked about how he didn't always like himself, didn't always love himself—but now he's among the best company. His is a time-less, ageless soul.

He has made a lot of friends over the years. A lot of people think it is very sad when they go to see a Hospice patient who is totally alone, because they have no family and have outlived all of their friends. That was the case with this man, but he wasn't sad. He was grateful. He said, "If it wasn't for this disease, I would never have met such incred-ible people, made such friends, met all these doctors, experienced all these things, and met you." I was amazed. He wasn't bitter at all. He was grateful for all of his life.

He also taught me something personal about the idea of marriage, because I never have gotten that right. I was married once, and I got real close to it about 40 other times, but chickened out.

He said, "You know, you have to change in order to be compatible with another person. That's life. And the older you get, the harder it is to change. So sometimes in order to preserve the friendship—so you don't resent the change so much—it is best to be alone or else you just keep trying to cram yourself together. It is a frustration, and you end up killing the friendship. So sometimes you make an active decision that it's best to just love a lot of people, and let them love you, and not have that mate idea—that one special person."

And I thought, *hmmm. Thank you for that insight.*

But this little man—who had no family and who had outlived his friends—sat there at the club surrounded by a group of people who loved him, young and old. He was there in his top hat and sunglasses. He got up on the stage. He did karaoke. He told jokes. And everybody turned around and paid attention to him. He had been doing this for 20 years. People just loved him.

When he came over and talked to me, people sensed what was going on. It is kind of unusual to invite your Hospice nurse to the bar with you, isn't it? But, I had to see what he did. I had to be sure it was really "him," and it was!

I realized something important: You can see people on the street, you can see them in different places and circumstances, and all of us make judgments. I had judged him! For all these years, I thought, "Oh, look at this poor little man." You know what I mean? And here he is—one of the kindest, most profound and spiritual human beings on the planet.

Anyway, he had his picture made with us because he loves to have his picture made with all of his friends. He said to me, "I'm going to miss this. I'm really going to miss it."

I said, "Mr. Green Jeans, you are not dead yet."

He said, "Yeah, but one thing that bothers me is that my legs keep falling out from under me."

I said, "You've got to use that cane that I got for you—that quadriceps cane, the four-prong one!"

He said, "Well, when I'm ready."

And I said, "Well, please just use it. Right when you feel like your legs are going to start giving out on you, start using it."

He said, "I think I'll know when that is."

I just thought to myself, I hope so. There was a raised stage and I thought his legs were going to buckle as he climbed up.

We all die—not to be depressing or anything. That isn't what this story is all about. But he has lived such a life of giving. He is not afraid. His spirit is very young.

RUSTY & VICTORIA

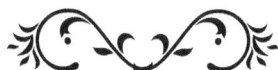

*T*his story has been the most difficult to tell, because of my continuing close relationship with Victoria's family. Victoria was the wife and caregiver for a patient that I had about four years ago. His name was Rusty. When I see her face I cry sometimes, because these folks were young and went through so much. Rusty was in his late 50's and Victoria was in her 40's.

Victoria asked me the other night what I wanted to tell you. What could I have possibly learned? I told her that what I learned—and I'll just give it to you in a nutshell right now—is that there are people who love their spouses enough to let go. They love them so much that they would rather lose them than see them in pain. I was reminded of all the things that people go through before they finally say, "Enough is enough. Let him be comfortable."

Victoria has been THE best role model for me on how to care for a loved one. Her children (she has two adult children) watched her as she took care of her husband—their stepfather. But let me get back to the beginning....

I was given Report on a man who had been diagnosed with cancer throughout his body —brain, lungs, gall bladder, stomach, etc. He lived in a very nice apartment. I found out later that these folks moved off of their sailboat when he was diagnosed as terminal. I didn't know what to expect, so, as I usually do, I prayed as I was walking up to the apartment. "God, just use me. Prepare them. Prepare me. And accomplish whatever You want. God...whatever."

When I walked in the door, I was shocked. Sitting there in a recliner was this man with white hair and a full white beard and he looked just like a Polar Bear. (I found out later that Victoria called him her Polar Bear.) He was a big guy. He was kind of sleepy, but alert enough to converse. I got the impression that this man needed to teach me something.

Victoria, was very intense—very intense. She listened to every word. She asked a lot of good questions. Her main questions were about the various medications. I told her about Hospice, about us being the liaison between the physician and the patient.

She was working at home for one of the local banks—they had allowed her to telecommute. She was a highly intelligent woman (you could just tell), and she was very realistic about Rusty's situation. Everything that I usually do for other patient caregivers, Victoria would do herself. She was young, wanted "to do it," and just assumed that she would. She was completely competent to take care of Rusty.

We discussed his medications. As we talked, he mentioned that she was giving him injections. Rusty had to be shot in the stomach with a needle every day. I just let that go for the first visit. I could tell it was a very sore subject. I gathered information from Rusty and Victoria; a lot had transpired in a short time. Later I found out that, even though Rusty's was a very short illness, there had been a lot of frustration throughout the process for both—especially Victoria. I felt my job was to get him (and the doctors) to the place where he didn't have to have any more treatments, tests, or pain.

I was learning how to dive and Rusty was a dive master. I was planning a trip to go diving for lobster, and he taught me how to wrap pantyhose around a "tickle stick," put this in a little hole, snag the lobster and pull him out. I believe on that visit I connected with Rusty. However, I could tell by his somewhat flat demeanor that his brain had been affected. This couple haunted me after I left.

During the next visit, Rusty was visibly weaker. He wasn't getting up very much. He had been nauseous and threw up.

I asked, "What did you do?"

She said, "I cleaned it up."

She later told me the rest of the story—Rusty was sitting in his recliner, and it was like Mount Vesuvius coming out of his mouth. It went all over her, the chair, the carpet and Rusty. She had held a giant bowl for him, but he missed the bowl entirely and it went everywhere, covering her from head to toe. As she turned around, her son Jacob came out to see what was going on. She said Jacob looked at her amazed face, and it was "everything he could do" not to laugh. She was still too surprised to react. She just went into the bathroom, got into the shower—clothes and all—and started laughing hysterically in the shower.

I thought, you know, if you can laugh through this—what a woman!

At this point, Jacob realized it was okay to laugh and began making jokes. Then he cleaned Rusty—and his beard, and his clothes, and his chair, and the carpet—with the ultimate tenderness and care, as if this were his very own flesh and blood.

On my second visit I talked to Victoria about the relationships that we at Hospice have with the physicians and how Hospice can actually intercede. Most youthful caregivers want to do everything possible to keep their loved one alive, regardless of their quality of life! Victoria asked me, "Do we have to keep doing all this—shots and pills, poking and probing?" His cancer was widespread. It was very clear he was dying and did not have much time.

I looked at her like she had lost her mind, because it was so unusual for a caregiver to ask me that question. I said, "No, WE at Hospice are about comfort and care."

I had talked to the Hospice physician about these shots that Rusty was getting. He said, "You know, he doesn't have to have those. He's not going to die a terrible death if he doesn't have them."

So I told Victoria she could make that choice. I told her she didn't have to give him any more shots. The expression her face took on was one of relief and gratitude. The kind of look that you get after you have been battling and battling and not sleeping and no one understands. And finally someone tells you: It's okay, you don't have to do this anymore. You can stop struggling. He does not have to be in any pain anymore.

She was very cool, calm, and collected, but the look on her face was—Thank you God! That's when we started talking about keeping Rusty comfortable through his eventual death.

Everything I suggested, Victoria did. Everything that would promote his comfort, Victoria tried. It was just incredible. I would call and say, "Hey, how are you doing?" and she would say, "Oh, I'm doing fine. You know he's getting weaker. He can't get up."

Most people would have been falling apart saying, "SEND THE NURSE! SEND THE NURSE!" That is the usual reaction, but Victoria knew this was to be expected. She understood the process. She was willing to let go.

I hadn't met Victoria's daughter at this point in time—Sarah. She was away at school. She is a special person. But I did meet Jacob, her son. Jacob is a writer and he wrote a piece about Rusty called, "Watching You Watch Me Die." Victoria gave me a copy of it and, after our visit, I went out in the parking lot, sat down on the sidewalk by my car, and read it. It was everything that they had gone through with the doctors and hospitals and Rusty's decline, and everything that Jacob had watched Rusty endure. I sat there on that curb and just sobbed.

People have to go through so much before they get to this moment—to where they are just so worn out, so tired of being probed and prodded and medicated, and told one more shocking thing, and forced to make one more life style change, and accept one more loss. It was absolutely incredible.

Jacob's story had a profound affect on me. I got him in contact with someone at Hospice, to check into publishing the story. I had a hospice physician read it, because I think that once you have been working in Hospice for a while, you forget that a person has really been through a lot by the time he or she becomes a Hospice patient. I know I can forget, so this was a very profound reminder.

On one of my last visits with Rusty, I was told that he was in his recliner almost full-time and very weak. We had a home health aide going in a couple of times a week to bathe him, but Victoria was doing the rest of the hands-on care, and she was still working at home. I was constantly amazed at how this woman would just laugh at herself and laugh at the extensive care that she needed to give and yet apply the seriousness required to accomplish what was needed. I have never seen anything like this.

The last time that I saw Rusty, he was in bed. He was in a coma and I was showing Victoria how to use the draw sheet. Anyway, we were turning him. Even after chemotherapy and radiation, Rusty was still a big guy.

She and I would talk and laugh, trying to work with him. Sometimes Victoria would laugh at the sheer absurdity of it all. Rusty had been so young and strong and healthy just a few months before. In order to do what you have to do, sometimes you just have to laugh to get through it.

The wild thing is that the people that you give the most to always want even more and are never satisfied—but I gave Victoria so little. She required so little assistance, and she was so grateful for every little hint. She was grateful for anything that made it easier for Rusty. These were very special people—very much in love.

When I left that day I knew that the time was close. I prepared Victoria as best I could by telling her that he would stop breathing, his heart would stop beating, and then she should call Hospice. I was very "cut and dried" with her, not because it was natural for me to be that way at the time. It was not. I was still sugarcoating things for other people, but she demanded bluntness.

I learned from this situation to always tell the truth and leave it up to the family to deal with the facts in their own way. The family members are the real heroes. Even though I have said this a million times already, I'll say it again. It's the caregivers actually taking care of their loved ones in their own homes who are the true heroes.

After Rusty died, Victoria and I became friends. She is one of the deepest people I've ever met and she has encouraged me to write this book. Victoria will never really understand what she gave me, but I'm telling you—it is more than I could possibly have given her.

There is more to this story… I might as well continue since I'm already crying…

About two years later Victoria's mom was in the hospital having surgery and was diagnosed with colon cancer. Victoria called me. She is the kind of friend with whom you just pick right up where you left off the next time you talk. Just the sound of Victoria's voice telling me about her mom let me know it was serious. After a short time, her mother ended up at a specialty hospital to recuperate from the surgery.

One day Victoria and I went shopping at a bookstore. We were talking about her mom. I don't know how it just came out of my mouth, but I said, "Victoria, it sounds like she's dying." I'm just so used to laying it out for Victoria, it seemed right.

She looked at me and she said, with no surprise, "It does, doesn't it!"

I was just stunned and amazed that God would prepare us both for this time by nurturing our friendship. That same day, while we were in the car, I said, "Let's go see your mom right now."

I could see at once that her mom was "out of it." Victoria told me that a dose of Ativan had knocked her out. The doctors were so concerned about this reaction that they cut back all her pain medications and stopped the Ativan immediately. Everybody thought the Ativan had knocked her out, but I was thinking—it sounds to me like she is trying to decline, but through human intervention she is being allowed to become uncomfortable.

Let me explain. Discomfort can cause a person's body to continue living even when they are supposed to die—THAT IS A FACT! With some people who are in pain, once they get comfortable—once they are finally medicated to where the pain goes away—their bodies can relax and they will let go. Similarly, if they are anxious people and their anxiety is controlled through medication or some other means, when that anxiety is controlled, they WILL let go. Victoria's mom was very anxious and in serious pain and discomfort.

When I left the hospital that day, I knew—Victoria knew—everybody knew that the time was close. Victoria had a long talk with her father that night. She had been "fighting" with the physicians, because they wanted to do more surgery and more tests. But her mom was so uncomfortable and just had so many other physical problems, it was clearly not a good course of action. So Victoria talked to her dad, and they both agreed—no more. They talked to her mom about it, and she totally agreed—no more.

I had met Victoria's daughter, Sarah, a few times during the last year. But it was during this time of crisis that I got a glimpse of her soul. This young woman was totally aware of what was going on. She was very supportive of her mother. Just the look in her eyes when we were talking about her grandmother endeared me to her forever. She was there for both Victoria and for her grandmother.

The next day I was off work, so I visited with Victoria and her mom. I saw that her mom was very uncomfortable. Victoria had requested the doctor to recommend Hospice care. However, Hospice didn't have a contract at that hospital, so they could not take care of her there. The physician was not comfortable ordering pain medication for this lady, but she WAS in pain.

There comes a time when I know that God puts me in places for a reason. At that point, I was beyond any fear of losing my job, so we went into action. Victoria and I had been through so much together. She was my friend, this patient needed help, and I knew I had to do something.

I called the Director of Nursing at Hospice, who is also a friend. I told her what was going on and that we needed to help. Of course, the Director was concerned that I was "working" at this hospital where there was no Hospice contract. I assured her I was not working, but just trying to help a friend. I asked her to please DO something!

My Director came through. She went over to the Assessment Referral Desk and talked to Lynnie and Martha, two very special people and great nurses. Lynnie called the doctor at the Hospital and got Victoria's mom some pain medication. She went that extra mile. Thank you, Lynnie!

Later I found out that Lynnie wanted to STRANGLE me for getting her involved in a very odd and strained situation! But, you know, I was just so appreciative. We have these little "compliment cards" at work. I filled out two and sent one to both Lynnie and Martha to say, "Thank you, thank you, thank you."

Even though I knew I was being a royal pain, it was more important for me to be the patient's advocate. It doesn't matter who the patient is or if they are assigned to me through Hospice. If a dying person is uncomfortable, I feel it is my place to be there for them. I don't want to be in pain when I'm at the end of MY life. Neither do I want my loved ones to be in pain at the end of their lives.

The assessment team arranged to get Victoria's mom home so she could be under Hospice care. They transferred her on a Friday, and I was on edge all day. I called Victoria. Her mom was heavily medicated and made the trip okay. Jacob rode in the ambulance with her, while Sarah and Victoria went ahead to prepare for her arrival. All the appropriate equipment was brought to the house, and a Hospice nurse completed an assessment.

As soon as Victoria's mom got home, apparently she declined very rapidly—and passed that same evening. Her family was all around her and handled everything just fine.

What really counts is how we help each other—our friends—our family. What counts is what we do for others. It's not our jobs. It's not financial security. It's not any of those things. It's doing the right thing and helping other people.

THE CAT LADY

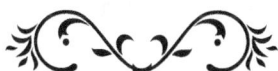

$\mathcal{I}$ met Blanche one afternoon after her admission to the Hospice program. She was only about 4 feet 11 inches tall. She had a big belly because of ovarian cancer, but she was up and around. She had all these dishes outside of her door with cat food in them. Blanche just loved animals. In fact, she loved animals more than she loved people.

Her son was a minister and her daughter-in-law was her main caregiver, but Blanche lived alone. She was very independent and I just loved her. My visits consisted of us getting to know each other. She was always grateful for everything I did.

Blanche had no short-term memory at all. She and I laughed about it, because we would be talking about something, she would write it on a sheet of paper (I had suggested she do this), and then she would set the paper down and forget where she put it. She must have had the Hospice phone number in seven different places in her house. Wherever you went, you would see all of these legal sheets with notes on them that she would write down to remember things. Blanche's attitude was that she might as well just enjoy the moment and laugh it off, because she couldn't remember anything, anyway!

We talked about how grateful we were that we didn't have a man to clean up after. She told me about her husbands and how she really loved living alone. She told me how Mitzie, her cat, was such good company. Mitzie didn't talk back. She didn't expect Blanche to look beautiful all the time, and she didn't expect Blanche to have the house clean all the time. Blanche was so real.

When Blanche found out that I was making wine as a hobby, she was very interested. She had a little something to drink every night, and she had this great bottle collection. They were beautiful bottles. She kept everything.

She had more boxes of "stuff" in her garage than anybody I had ever seen. That is, outside of a guy I dated one time that couldn't even walk into his apartment, because he had boxes up to the ceiling. But that's not our story here.

Blanche was just a trip! Her daughter-in-law would get upset because she would write these giant checks using money that she didn't have. She would order things out of magazines, like pillows to go on her couch, crystal goblets, whatever. The daughter-in-law would get very concerned, too, because Blanche couldn't remember if she had written a check or not, or for what amount.

As time went on, Blanche's left leg began to swell. The hospital ran tests, but found no clot. We put her on some extra diuretics[31]. This seemed to help at first, but then she couldn't remember to take them.

Six months passed and Blanche's condition did not decline, so she decided that she wanted to go back to the doctor and have some aggressive treatment. Our visits came to an end, and I "inactivated" her from the Hospice program.

Becoming a Hospice "flunky" is a good thing. All we have to do is inactivate a person from their Hospice benefits, and they can go and seek aggressive treatment. Later on, if they start declining, they can come back in the program. They just need a doctor to refer them back to Hospice and be readmitted.

Months after Blanche left Hospice, I got the phone call saying that she had started to decline and was returning to the program. When I went to see her, she barely made it to the door and then went right back to the couch. Her belly was so big, her leg was still large and she was incredibly weak. She still had her great sense of humor and she remembered me. None of her hair had come out from the treatments. It was still just this beautiful, soft gray. It was only an inch long, but it was so pretty.

Blanche had had a spiritual awakening during her time away from Hospice, and she was okay with dying. She still had no short-term memory, which was just hysterical, because I was so stressed that mine was going, too. Our visits were just filled with laughter.

Blanche grew very weak. One day I called her at 3:00 in the afternoon, and she was still in bed. She had very little breath. She had consented to use oxygen, but she didn't want a home health aide to come in, because she kept crazy hours. I didn't want to inconvenience her, because this was her life.

Ultimately, she got to the point that she was so weak she couldn't get out of bed. I went to her house and met her daughter-in-law. Blanche was too weak to get out of bed, so I lay in bed beside her. The daughter-in-law was sitting on the side of the bed.

I said, "Blanche, honey, you can't be alone anymore. I hate to be the person who tells you that, but that time has come."

She looked at me, and said, "I know, and I really appreciate you telling me. I'll just do whatever is easiest for my family."

I encouraged her daughter-in-law to go see the Hospice Center, because Blanche didn't want anyone to stay in her home. She had been alone for so long that any person in her home would have felt like an invasion. I was very sensitive to this, because I knew Blanche well from the time I had spent with her, and I knew she felt very strongly about that.

Blanche's son and daughter-in-law went to look at the center. There was a bed available, so we had an ambulance take her to the Hospice Center that afternoon. That was a miracle, as beds are not usually available that fast.

When Blanche arrived at the Hospice Center, I got her tucked in and sat with her for a minute. The look on her face was one of gratitude and love. It was as if she and I had marched through this process together, and it was finally time to let a good friend go. I was so glad that she was at peace, comfortable, and in a safe place.

She had made a long journey with this process, and it just gave me complete confidence in our God. He takes the most independent people that have the strongest will to live, and when it's their time, He gives them peace when they ask for it.

She looked at me, and said, "I want to thank you for everything that you have done for me—our laughter—and our visits. You have really been a big part of my life."

Her daughter-in-law walked in at that point, and Blanche said, "And THAT young lady. I don't call her a daughter-in-law. I call her my daughter."

It was a special moment. God was using this to bring everybody together and give us an understanding that we were truly loved.

As I hugged Blanche goodbye for the last time, I said to her, "You know, when you cross over, my best friend Eleanor will be waiting for you. She's going to welcome you. It will be very good."

She said, "Oh, I know it will be."

She was tired, so I told her I would let her rest and keep everybody out. Her main concern about going to the Hospice Center was that she would have so many people in and out. So I told the staff that she wanted to be alone.

After the nurse did her initial assessment, Blanche went to asleep. We kicked everybody out of the room and I left, knowing it was the last time I would see this tremendous woman. However, I knew that she wasn't really alone. She and God were so close.

Blanche died shortly after that. I talked to the daughter-in-law on the phone and everyone was okay. It was a good experience for that family, as they developed such closeness at the end.

Blanche gave me a lot. She taught me that when your short-term memory leaves (as mine surely will) that you can still love and be lovable. She taught me that you can still have worth and that you can be a viable living creature who can help other people. She helped me and her family in ways that we'll never totally understand.

This was such an incredible journey. I think about it a lot. I think about how some of my dearest friends are now with Eleanor.

MAGGIE

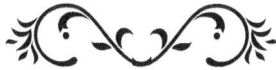

When I first met Maggie Wilde, I found her to be delightful—just delightful. Maggie had acute leukemia, and the main issue was her blood transfusions. With this kind of disease process it's difficult because eventually the transfusions stop being effective. The patient grows weaker and more tired, and struggles to the hospital for transfusions, hoping for some improvement for a short time. Usually, I'm the one who has to tell the patient and the family that it's not working anymore.

It's just very ugly, and I was not looking forward to going through this with Maggie.

However, her personality overcame my reluctance, because she was just...well, a "wild woman." She always dressed and looked great. She had a mad sense of humor. Oh, my gosh! She had the humor of a red-head.

On my first visit with her, she was in bed. Of course, she was very tired, as is typical of leukemia. Her husband always sat on the other side of the bed. They were in their late 70's and lived in a big house with their grown daughter, Julie, who became one of my friends. Julie was a dynamic woman.

I went to their house toward the end of the day, because of their schedule and my routing. Maggie would usually get home from the hospital at 2:00 P.M. after having her transfusions, so I would always schedule our appointments later in the day. I always left feeling better than when I got there. I'd be sitting there talking to her about her health, and she was so willing to talk and, to add humor to the situation, I'd leave there just flying high. It was great.

In retrospect, I think God knew what He was doing when He later moved me into PRN during this time, because I just couldn't imagine being objective enough to be effective during Maggie's final days. I couldn't even picture that, because I got so close to this family.

The kids just LOVED their parents. Julie would call me, and say, "Well, WHY is Momma's body doing this?"

I would call "Dr. Tennis" to discuss the situation. Pretty soon, they got to know that Dr. Tennis and I could work pretty well together. Dr. Tennis and I started calling Maggie, "our baby." The family loved that...they just loved that.

Eventually, I started answering Julie's questions by saying, "Okay, medically this is what you do, but if it were MY mom and I was taking care of her at home, I would also do THIS or do it THIS WAY...."

Julie understood and approved. I dealt with Maggie as if she were my mom and her family were my family. This made it easy, while her symptoms were under control.

Whenever her hemoglobin counts (her blood levels) would be low, she needed transfusions. At first her blood transfusions were every three weeks. Then they became more frequent, about every 10 days.

Maggie starting getting even weaker, and she became very short of breath. Getting oxygen into her home was difficult, since Maggie saw oxygen as a defeat. I had to baby her into it. I said, "Listen, just humor me. I would feel better if you had oxygen in the house to use when your blood counts get so low that you get short of breath. That shortness of breath happens because you don't have enough oxygen floating through your body."

So she agreed. She used it, but she just HATED it. She loved life and did not want to leave or be more restricted.

Transfusions were soon required every seven days, and she got weaker and weaker. She started getting confused and was hallucinating. She did eventually come out of that, but before she did I convinced the family that she was declining and would need a hospital bed for easier care. She really appeared to be declining.

About three days after this period of confusion, I went back to see her. She was nearly lucid again. When Maggie and I were alone in the room, she told me, "You know, it really bothers me, to hallucinate." She went on, "And it wasn't just like I'm feeling out of control either, there is something more to it."

Then she told me about her mom, who had Alzheimer's. She had been with her mom towards the end, and her mom did some crazy things. I realized that Maggie was afraid that she had Alzheimer's and this was what made her so upset about hallucinating.

She wasn't hurting anybody and it was no problem for the family. Actually, she was downright likable when she was hallucinating! You know…some people can be pleasantly confused, and she was one of those people. But the root of her fear was that she might end up being a screaming, out-of-control person like her mother had been toward the end. Her mom had been just a totally beautiful woman, but when she got Alzheimer's, she wasn't the same. Maggie was very afraid of being like that.

We had a lot of discussions, Maggie and I, on the spiritual level I guess we were kind of alike inside, on some of the spiritual things.

She said things that I had never heard other people talk about. One day she said, "You know the family wants me to talk about funeral arrangements. And I think for space reasons and everything, I really should be cremated. But I have this real fear that they will be putting my body into the incinerator, and I will wake up and not be dead. I have a terror of not being dead when I leave this house."

I've never heard anybody actually say that before, but I have that same exact fear. And that became a very chief point for her towards the end of her life. I promised her I would make sure she was definitely dead before the funeral home took her body out of the house.

Well, Maggie's health improved, and she looked at me one day and said, "Would you do one thing for me?"

"What's that?" I asked.

"Would you get that darned hospital bed out of my room?" she said. "It makes me feel like I'm going to DIE at any moment!"

"Okay, no problem," I said.

So we took the hospital bed out, and she hovered along for a while. She didn't have a lot of energy. She wasn't declining, but she didn't get up and move around very much. With her particular disease process, her tissues swelled quite a bit, so she was really uncomfortable getting up on her feet.

Her family kept calling Triage, saying, "Her left leg is swollen. Her left leg is swollen." Then somebody would go over on the weekend to take care of it. On Monday I would hear about it. But by the time I would get there, her leg wouldn't be swollen at all, because they would have had her elevate it. Triage would always check her for a clot, but there was no evidence of a clot.

During a visit, I noticed her leg hanging off the side of her bed, and I asked her, "Do you sleep like that?"

She said, "Yeah, I guess I do."

I said, "That's why your leg is swollen all the time!"

It was so funny. She just couldn't believe that it was so simple. When I told Triage, they were hysterical. Her leg is hanging off the bed and that's why we've been sending our people over there looking for blood clots!?

Another lesson—when people are terminally ill we tend to assume the worst, when it may be something very simple causing a problem. In this case, she just had an extremity that was hanging lower than the other parts of her body.

Then Maggie started to decline again—not the same as the first time, but she got extremely weak. One day I was over talking to her, when her husband stood up and walked towards the bathroom past the oxygen machine. All of a sudden he started scrambling to avoid falling. Then he tripped and exclaimed, "Oh God, help me!"

I didn't know what was happening, but I got up trying to catch him. Maggie sprang out of bed to go help him, like I've never seen her move before. The man was going down by the corner of this little wooden area that would have cracked his head open. There was no way that his head should have missed that area—I still don't understand to this day how he missed it. He fell and everything crashed. I was just thinking... Oh God, help us...God, help us!

By this time, Maggie had definitely sprung to life. She was on the floor with her husband. I was looking at the back of his head for bleeding, because there was no way that this man could have NOT busted his head open. I saw his head going right towards that corner, but I couldn't find any blood. I looked at his pupils and I talked to him. He was a little bit out of it, and we couldn't get him off the floor. I took his blood pressure, and it was really low—60/40. I checked his heart rate, and it was 20! I'm thinking, No, No, No, No—YOU are NOT the one who is supposed to be dying here!

I took his blood pressure again—it was 70/50, and I thought...this man's heart is giving out. I gave a little cardio thump on his pericardium. After that, he started to revive. I rolled him onto his knees and actually got him onto the bed. I took his blood pressure again—it was 80/60. His heart rate was up to 30 this time. It was NOT good, but he began to come around. I got him something to drink, and Maggie was still up and walking around the house like I've never seen her walk around before. She had just SPRUNG to LIFE.

I talked to Mr. Wilde, trying to stay calm, assessing the situation.

He said, "Yeah, they've been trying to get me to put a pacemaker in now for two years, but you know, Maggie got sick, and I kind of put it off."

I thought...You TELL me this NOW!

We called his cardiologist, who said it was time for him to come in. By this time, Maggie was DRESSED. She didn't look like the sick one at all. We called Julie and got him to the cardiologist.

Julie called me that night saying, "Dad's been admitted to the hospital. They are going to put a pacemaker in tomorrow."

The next day, I called Julie. She told me they couldn't put the pacemaker in, because he was on a high dose of Coumadin[32]. This meant that if he HAD hit his head, he probably would have bled to death. I am convinced that when he yelled, "God, help me" as he fell, that God heard him, allowing him to avoid the fatal corner.

I went to see him at the hospital when he was ready for the surgery. Maggie was there every day! People there wondered which one was the Hospice patient. They just couldn't believe it was Maggie—her color and strength improved. She just looked like the supportive wife. In fact, I started to wonder if she was ill at all!

Mr. Wilde did get the pacemaker, and he went home from the hospital in a few days. The next week, when I went to visit, his color was back to normal. Before, he had appeared a bit pasty-looking, but now he seemed healthy.

Maggie had forgotten she was sick, and she went into remission. That's the only way I can explain it. Her remission lasted a good month. I think that people rise to the occasion for their loved ones. These people are very spiritual and I knew God really worked it out for them.

It was at this time that I went up to North Carolina to take care of my dad after his surgery. I was talking to my mom about my Hospice work. I told her I thought I was getting burned out, because I could no longer put any barriers up. I wanted to crawl into bed with these people and die with them. It was getting too intense. So, when I returned to Florida, I left full-time nursing and went PRN. It was a good thing, as I was worried about becoming less effective.

Another nurse took over my patients, including Maggie, but I still kept track of this family from a distance. They understood it and felt good since Dr. Tennis still had a relationship with them. Even the nurses knew they didn't have to give Dr. Tennis a lot of information when they called him, since he knew Maggie and her history pretty well.

About one month after I went PRN, I was working Triage on a Sunday and got a call from the Wilde family. Actually I got a call from the runner, because Maggie was pretty non-responsive and the runner was at her home. The runner had talked to Dr. Tennis and was told to stop Maggie's Ativan unless she became restless.

Julie had called me back later and said, "Mom's getting restless again. What do we do?"

I said, "Well, I'll put it this way. If she is non-responsive and gets restless, this may be the restlessness that comes on right before you die. If you give her Ativan and she relaxes, she will probably go on. You need to be ready for that and you need to tell your dad that, too."

Julie gave her mom the Ativan and called me back in an hour. She said, "Mom is very calm. She is not restless now."

Maggie and I had discussed her fear of the dying process earlier and I had assured Maggie she would not have pain. I told her that we had supplied her with all the medications she would need so that she would be comfortable. Julie and Mr. Wilde knew of her fears and wanted to ensure her comfort as well.

By this time they had already called the family in twice, because she had almost died twice. But she kept reviving, so nobody really believed her anymore. It was like the boy who cried wolf.

Then I got a call at 6:45 that same evening. It was from Mr. Wilde. He said, "Patty, she's gone."

I said, "Okay, how is everybody?"

And he said, "We are okay. We're fine. She wasn't restless. She didn't suffer. She just went on." He said that he was lying next to her in bed. They were all prepared.

Mr. Wilde told me later that the Triage nurse had suggested to the family that day that they get a hospital bed. Mr. Wilde said, "I KNOW that's why she left today, because she DIDN'T want that DARN hospital bed in the room!" He had such a great sense of humor.

It was a miracle that I was on Triage that day. Since I couldn't get out there until eight o'clock, I sent Chaplain Woods out to verify the death. But I needed to go there myself. I think I wanted to say goodbye to her—not so much that I thought her spirit was still there. I just needed some closure.

The chaplain had put his hand on her carotid artery and verified death, but I wanted to fulfill my promise to Maggie. That promise was that I would do every test that I could do to make sure that she was gone before she was taken out of the house, and I intended to fulfill that promise.

When I got to the house, Chaplain Woods was counting the medications. I went into the bedroom—and there was Maggie. Her mouth was wide open, her head up on the pillows. Her leg was hanging off the side of the bed, like always. Everyone was peaceful and calm. I tried to close her mouth, but it wouldn't close. It was like cement. She had been dead about two hours. I kept pushing her chin, to get it closed, because it really does upset the families when the mouth is wide open. As hard as I tried to close it, it wouldn't budge.

I decided it was time to do the examination. So I looked over at her body and started walking towards her to take her blood pressure, check her heart rate, etc. I thought I saw her chest rise and fall like she was breathing. I said to myself, okay, this is not real. I know about these things—they play with your head. You think the person is alive when they are not, because you stare at them too long.

Then Julie came over and said, "Oh, did you see her foot! Her foot just moved!"

I wanted to say—Yeah, yeah, I'm having visual hallucinations too, Julie! But I didn't want to unnerve her, so instead I mumbled, "Hmm…Okay…."

I took Maggie's blood pressure—nothing. That was fine. I checked the carotid artery and the radial artery. I felt nothing. Then I took my stethoscope and put it on the apex of the heart. I thought I HEARD something. Listening—listening—no, I didn't hear anything. I felt around, and I went to each part of the heart. I listened, and it was very, very quiet in the room. People were just going about their business. I listened hard, and then it became painfully clear to me that I was not hearing a darn thing. I heard nothing.

It was then that I just totally lost it, and I cried for a good solid five minutes. This was so hard, because I had a great relationship with

Maggie. I would miss her—so many people would miss her. And to see her body void of life, my denial was crucified, and I kind of collapsed.

Finally, I was able to compose myself. Julie went out and poured me a glass of wine and brought it in to me. A Catholic nun, who had visited Maggie a few times, was also there. When she asked for an Irish Cream, I knew it would be okay to drink. I wasn't on duty, so I could sit there and drink with the nun. I knew Maggie would think that was pretty funny.

Another weird thing happened. Mr. Wilde was lying next to Maggie pretty much the whole time and he kept saying "Is her mouth closing?"

"You know, Mr. Wilde, I had that same reaction." I said. "No, Hon, her mouth isn't really closing, but I do understand." And I told him about how I saw her chest rise and fall and everything. And I told him how our imaginations really do weird things.

Then I walked over towards the side of the bed and saw that her mouth had closed almost all the way shut and her face looked normal! Now, gravity doesn't do this. Rigor mortis does NOT do this. I have been around many dead people for hours, and I have NEVER seen this happen. Her mouth had closed. She looked just like she did when she was alive.

I looked over at Mr. Wilde and I said, "Her mouth... Her mouth did close. I can't explain this."

Chaplain Woods needed to destroy the medications, so he took all the pills and dumped them into a big bowl to take to the toilet for flushing. The chaplain and I were in the bathroom, and I started to laugh. Everything became very funny. Julie came into the bathroom, and she thought everything was funny too. We were sitting in the bathroom holding our stomachs, laughing hysterically over having to wait for this toilet to flush while pouring the medications in. It looked like a bowel of porridge or something with all those pills. Hospice humor is sick humor, to be sure, but that is just how we cope sometimes.

I kept my promise to Maggie—I absolutely made sure that she was dead before anyone took her away. And that she would not like wake up all of a sudden right before she was to be cremated. And that was so cool—that she shared that with me.

Now Maggie was just as much of a priss as I am, so Julie and I put a little rouge and a nice shade of lipstick on her so she would be presentable to her sons. I was about to leave, as it was getting towards midnight, and I was really tired.

Then Julie said that we should paint her nails. She said, "Momma always wanted that. She always wanted her nails perfect when she left the house. She never liked to leave without everything in order." So we filed and polished her nails and made sure she looked pristine.

Maggie was like a mother and sister to me. She included me in her family just naturally. She shared her most intimate thoughts with me. That experience made me a better nurse, and a better person. Thank you, Maggie.

Epilogue

It is sixteen days after the act of terrorism on the World Trade Center and the Pentagon—year 2001. I am sitting in a meditation garden in North Carolina writing this epilogue with so few words to express what I want to say.

While writing this book I was very aware of a grief cycle that happens with the patient and the family and the Hospice worker when someone is terminally ill and dies. But now I am witnessing and experiencing the grief cycle of a nation, along with every other person who lives in the United States. We have lost people. We have lost a sense of safety. We have lost concepts. We have lost the fantasy that this country is a safe place to live. This country, the whole world, is grieving.

It makes me realize even more the lessons that have come through in the preceding stories, which are the need for getting to know God one-on-one as a person—you and God—because life can be very short. Tell the people you love that you love them—you may not have a chance tomorrow, so do it now. Be good to people and be forgiving.

I am reminded especially of how truly difficult it is to understand that life and death are a process and so many things are out of our control. The process is living, and loving, and letting go of the things and of the people you love. Resting after they are gone, healing, and going through the frustration of trying to move on. That feeling of being unable to function because nothing is the same any more, and you move three steps forward and two steps back. It is a process, and you will come through it. Life goes on.

These past sixteen days have given me a whole new perspective on grieving—the grief cycle, and the process. I realize even more profoundly what the Hospice families, and the patients themselves, go through on a daily basis. It has renewed my respect and admiration for them, as well as every person in the United States. The people who go through this, those who do what they need to do to take care of the people that they love, are going through a whole new dimension of life. They are heroes, as well as those who have died.

I don't know if I will be staying in Hospice in some capacity or moving on. I have learned to leave that decision in God's hands. I really wish that I could hug each of you who read this and just let you know that you are not alone. There is a God that loves us so intensely and so individually, and you can find Him when you feel alone, when you feel so frustrated and you don't feel connected with people or anything on this planet—there really is a Master Connector.

That is the only one thing I am sure of right in this red hot moment, in the middle of the mountains and the forest in North Carolina, and that is that God IS, and that the more you cry and the more depth of sorrow that you can feel, the more joy you can also feel.

God bless you.

Index

— L —

Laughter. *See* humor. *See* humor. *See* humor
Laxative
  Haley's MO, 45
  Senokot, 14
Legacies, 108

— M —

Morphine, 52, 75, 103

— N —

Nausea Relief Medication
  Phenergan, 61
Near-death Experience, 108
Nutritional Liquid Food Supplement
  Ensure, 71

— P —

P.A.. *See* Physician's Assistant
Pamphlet. *See* Signs and Symptoms of Dying Process
Parkinson's Medication
Sinemet, 15
Physician's Assistant, 38
Pranks. *See* humor
Prayer, 80
PRN, 68,107

— R —

Release Excess Fluids from Body
  Diurese, 82
Religious Conversion, 28
Remission of Cancer, 93
Risk Assessments, 52

Endnotes

Chapter One

[1] A laxative

[2] A medication to treat Parkinson's symptoms

Chapter Two

[3] 2 Corinthians 5:8

[4] Medical/Surgical – for surgical patients

Chapter Three

[5] A nursing term for the information about a patient

[6] An anti-psychotic medication

[7] A drug often prescribed for anxiety, which can also be used for shortness of breath, or nausea and vomiting.

[8] Physician's Assistant

[9] An indwelling tube in the bladder attached to a drainage bag.

[10] To be taken every six to eight hours, as needed.

[11] A medication to assist in taking water out of the body.

Chapter Four

[12] A protective patch put on broken down skin.

[13] An anti-inflammatory

[14] Do Not Resuscitate order

[15] I have no idea how to spell this, but that's how it sounds!

[16] Sustained release morphine every twelve hours

Chapter Five

[17] Test to show abnormalities of the cervix

[18] A nutritional liquid food supplement

[19] The term used for that end-of-life breathing

[20] A medication, generally given for restlessness, which has other uses, such as for nausea relief.

[21] Anti-nausea medications

[22] Another medication used for nausea

[23] Give her a diuretic to release the excess fluids from her body.

[24] Due to liver enlargement, this makes the abdomen area very large.

[25] Depends® is a brand name of adult diapers

Chapter Six

[26] Laxatives

[27] Bleed out could happen if a lung tumor grows into a major artery. If this occurs, blood can come out of the mouth, nose, or ears. The person dies quickly and painlessly. The only "pain" a patient may have is if they see panic on the face of the caretakers. I recommend the family purchase dark towels and sheets, and if it occurs to sit with the patient, wipe his or her mouth, and don't panic.

[28] Gave up eating.

[29] A sheet under the patient that allows for turning and bathing the patient more easily.

[30] A nurse on as-needed status, rather than full-time

[31] To reduce fluids

[32] A blood thinning medication

About the Author

*P*atricia Blunt Weatherford, RN, has spent ten years serving others during the most intimate time of their lives. With her passion for interacting with people, she brings awareness to the community through seminars and classes. This often-avoided issue is explored by adding humor to an important subject once considered taboo.

She educates hospice professionals in clinical skills, assessment, and family dynamics in the dying process. Weatherford is a personal trainer in Stress Management and facilitates programs on Wellness through Nutrition, Exercise and Meditation.

As her first book, *Eleanor's Gift* has been very successful, and a second book on the year after is in the making. Patty lives with her husband in Midlothian, Virginia.

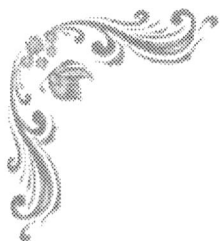

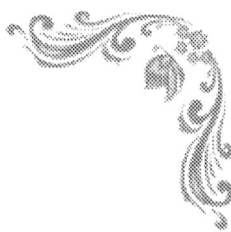

To order copies of *Eleanor's Gift*

or

to schedule speaking engagements,
email author
Patricia Blunt Weatherford
at
eleanorsgift@aol.com

Copies of *Eleanor's Gift* may be purchased for $15.95 each,
plus $3.00 shipping and handling for the first copy.
S & H is $1.00 per book for each additional copy.

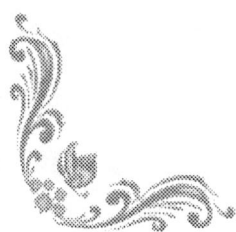

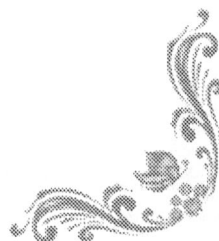

www.ingramcontent.com/pod-product-compliance
Lightning Source LLC
Chambersburg PA
CBHW031853090426
42741CB00005B/466